DEATH IN SLOW MOTION

A Memoir of a Daughter, Her Mother, and the Beast Called Alzheimer's

Eleanor Cooney

Perennial

An Imprint of HarperCollins*Publishers*

A hardcover edition of this book was published in 2003 by HarperCollins Publishers.

HarperCollins books may be purchased for educational, business, or sales promotional use. For information please write: Special Markets Department, HarperCollins Publishers Inc., 10 East 53rd Street, New York, NY 10022.

First Perennial edition published 2004.

Designed by Jeffrey Pennington

The Library of Congress has catalogued the hardcover edition as follows:

Cooney, Eleanor.
Death in slow motion: my mother's descent into Alzheimer's / Eleanor Cooney. —1st ed.
p. cm.
ISBN 0-06-621396-7
1. Cooney, Eleanor V. 2. Alzheimer's disease—Patients—Biography.
3. Alzheimer's disease—Patients—Family relationships.
4. Mothers and daughters. I. Title.

RC523.2.C665 2003
362.1'96831'0092—dc21 [B]
2002068935

ISBN 0-06-093797-1 (pbk.)

04 05 06 07 08 ❖/RRD 10 9 8 7 6 5 4 3 2 1

Praise for *Death in Slow Motion*

"A strong and honest book."   —Lewis Lapham, *Harper's* magazine

"Stunning and eloquent in its wounded passion."   —*Chicago Tribune*

"Wry, learned prose."   —*Time* magazine

"A novelist who has written books set in ancient China, Cooney writes a stark prose that is vivid, riveting, and stylish. She keeps the reader hooked by also writing about her mother's remarkable life. . . . There are anecdotes of growing up in Connecticut that Cooney likens to a John Cheever story, in which characters are driven by demons to illicit behavior."   —*Philadelphia Inquirer*

"Cooney tells it all with a fine and rare mix of black humor and bleak honesty."   —*Kirkus Reviews*

"Poignant. . . . Terrific. . . . Consider it a must-read."   —*Booklist*

"Well-written [and] harrowing."   —*Publishers Weekly*

"Grim, heart-wrenching, luminous, tender, and terrifying."   —*BookStreet USA*

"Crackles with grim humor and pragmatism."   —*St. Louis Post-Dispatch*

"Savagely detailed, no-holds-barred. . . . She tells her story with panic-stricken speed and wicked black humor . . . immensely moving and terrifyingly funny. The writing remains vibrant and compelling throughout. Imagine listening to a talented war correspondent's account of a hopeless and heroic battle—Cooney has done nothing less."   —*San Francisco Chronicle*

"A harrowing portrait. . . . A shockingly frank and passionately written memoir. . . . The reader might not be able to bear the truth of this book without Cooney's own special brand of black humor."   —*Tulsa World*

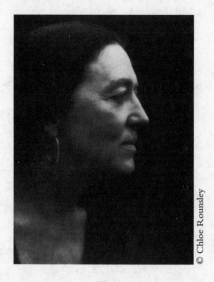

© Chloe Rounsley

About the Author

ELEANOR COONEY has published four novels.
She lives in Mendocino, California.

For Mike and Mary

ACKNOWLEDGMENTS

First, my huge thanks and gratitude to the ones who quite literally made this book possible: Lewis Lapham, Gail Winston and Lisa Queen. And for help and support before, during and after, a thousand thanks to Christine Walsh, Chloe Rounsley, Drew Sparks, Mitchell Clogg III, John Bellinger and J.P. Struthers. And a thousand more thanks to my heroines, Jenny Johnson of Redwood Caregivers Resource Center, and Melanie Richardson, formerly of Summerfield House. And of course, to my heroes: Mitch, Tommy, Allen.

CONTENTS

DEATH IN SLOW MOTION

All was well, for what was dust had when living been loved.

—Nelson Algren

CHAPTER ONE

God Is a Murderer

September: About eleven months since we moved my mother to California to live with us, I wake at dawn from queasy dreams where I'm sliding down steep slimy banks of mucky pools or flying in a crowded flimsy airplane being pulled to earth by heavy gravity or searching for lost kittens in a dank primeval forest. The morning light is gray and hopeless; I hear my mother's feet outside shuffling like the Swamp Thing across the driveway to get her morning paper. Her presence pulls umbilically at my gut. I gulp a Valium and burrow under the blankets, my body stiff with fear and fatigue, head throbbing from too much wine the night before. Though the room is still, I can feel acceleration in my stomach, my bed a rollercoaster car just cresting and starting its plunge, but the acceleration is not of motion, it's of time, warp-speeding me into my own old age and decrepitude. The thoughts that seethe around in my brain are pornographically mortal. They shock even me.

Whoever said love is stronger than death was full of malarkey. There's no contest. Death is a sumo wrestler, and it slams love to the mat every time. When my mother's husband died twelve years ago, her own life was pretty much sucked out of her, though she still walks and talks. I loved Mike, too. Let me give you some advice: Unless you have deep religious faith (I have none at all) or objective detachment bordering on the abnormal, don't read the autopsy report of someone you loved. I peeked at a few pages of Mike's, and regret it. There are no euphemisms there. Bone saws and steel buckets will remind you just how strong death really is.

And death's warm-up act, Alzheimer's, is no less a brute. You'll never be the same once it's paid you a visit—believe me. Just a short time ago, I was ignorant. I'd heard stories, of course, but like winning the lottery or going to prison or being abducted by aliens, you just can't know how it is until you've lived it. Now I know. Alzheimer's is death in slow motion, and it has the ability to kill love while the person you love still breathes.

My mother was always my favorite person. And a lot of other people's, too. Hip, cool, brilliant, funny, sane. A writer. My ultimate confidante and sympathizer. Not like the other mothers. My friends always came to my house to escape their regular boring (or crazy) parents. I have a picture of me and a bunch of teenaged friends one summer in the mid-sixties cavorting in the backyard of the house in Connecticut, my mother sitting in our midst in a canvas chair, slim elegant blue-jeaned legs crossed, laughing. We're all free and easy, horsing around, performing for her. She's in her early forties, beautiful, probably a year or so away from meeting Mike.

She was born in 1922. The first shadows fell around 1997 with blanks in her short-term retention and disquietingly uncharacteristic lapses in judgment. It's plain to us now that she struggled to hide it for a couple of years. She's graduated to delusions and disorientation and now some long-term memory loss, too.

My mother's been severely, profoundly depressed since Mike's death, and I believe that this was the cause of her mental deterioration. I don't have hard, irrefutable clinical evidence that this is so—it's just what I *know*. I believe protracted despair weakened her, changed the physical structure of her brain, made her vulnerable to the disease. Chronic sorrow is a parasite. It eats your strength, appropriates your will, moves like toxic sludge through every system of the mind and body. And my theory is not so farfetched. Everyone knows that depression compromises the immune system. Look at the statistics on cancer survival and mental health. How often do we hear about couples dying within weeks or days of each other? Alzheimer's is still a mystery, but they're slowly finding things out. Recent research points to an autoimmune disorder—an inflammation of the brain. So there it is. I think grief literally burned out the circuits of my mother's brain.

And it did it in a sly, self-serving way that points to itself as the culprit: It robbed her of her wit, intellect, judgment and competence, but it made sure its own pathways were sturdy and intact. She forgot everything, but she didn't forget her grief. It stayed vital, grew stronger, gathered momentum. If I'm completely wrong, and my mother was going to lose her memory even if Mike hadn't died, her illness would not have taken the form that it did, fueled by heartache and vodka, shaped by desolation. None of this would have happened.

But Mike did die. And it did happen.

In mid-November 1989, late in the afternoon, my mother and brother and I filed into the Intensive Care Unit of a major San Diego hospital. We stood in awe around Mike's bed. He was just coming out of the anesthesia after a major and radical six-hour operation where they'd opened up his chest and put him on a heart-lung machine. This had not been bypass surgery or anything else we've all heard of. This was such a rare, specialized and risky procedure that only two hospitals in the country performed it. I'd never seen an I.C.U. before. It was a temple of mystery with its hushed atmosphere, brilliant lights and stupefyingly sophisticated technology, Mike's bed the altar where human sacrifices were offered to a perverse deity with a jaded appetite.

Mike struggled to focus. He grasped at our hands. My mother kissed him and spoke in his ear. He'd made it. All of us, Mike included, thought that if he died it would be on the table. But he'd come through and opened his eyes. He was out of danger.

Wrong. He was fully conscious for eleven days, during which he went from believing he'd made it to knowing he wouldn't. To knowing he'd be leaving my mother a widow at age sixty-seven. Unable to talk because of the respirator down his throat. On the day of his death, I had a genuine psychic premonition, something I'm not prone to at all. I heard my mother's voice just before the phone rang.

Mike was husband Number Three, twelve years younger than she, the love of her life. When they got together in 1966, he was thirty-two and she was forty-four. He was fifty-five when he died. Real heartbreak is another of those things you have to experience to fully appreciate. His death broke my heart, and it shredded my mother's. Just about everyone in the town where they lived was devastated. The mentally slow woman who sorted recyclables at the local market threw an armload of cans onto the floor when someone told her Mike had died. Her face crumpled, and she cried, right there in the store. "That nice Mr. Harwood," she said. Hundreds of people came to his memorial service and tore their hair. I'd never seen anything like it. And we, his family and friends, weren't the only ones who lost. The world lost, too. Michael Harwood was an important environmental activist and author getting ready to write his magnum opus. He had a mountain of research and notes all ready to go. My mother held on to those files and books and papers for years, as if maybe, just maybe, they could lure Mike back from the dead . . .

Mike was about as different from my mother's first two husbands as the first two husbands were different from each other. Husband Number Two, Tim Durant, my first stepfather, was a dashing, charming prick who ran with a glamorous crowd, including the likes of John Huston, José Ferrer and Charlie Chaplin. She married him on Huston's estate in County Kildare in 1954. I have a newspaper clipping from the *Irish Times*, a photograph of Huston kissing her at the wedding, Durant in full formal fox-hunting attire, grinning, nobly handsome, my mother young and gorgeous and deliriously happy.

Deliriously happy is what the marriage emphatically turned out not to be. She told us once that a few minutes after that picture was taken, Durant was up on his thoroughbred, about to gallop off to the ta-ra of the hunting horn, when he leaned down and said to his new bride: Let's keep in touch.

Uh-oh, she thought. And she was right.

But Durant was not entirely without redeeming qualities. He's the guy who bought the house she still lived in—for seven grand in 1955, cheap even then. Plus he provided her with the terrific pen name of Mary Durant and a great fictional character: She laid him bare like a frog on the dissection tray, disguising him as Hoyt Bentley in her 1963 masterpiece, *Quartet in Farewell Time.*

And my father? He wasn't a prick at all. He was a handsome Irishman, tall and strapping with curly black hair, a scholar and a quiet genius, a New York City boy who'd never driven a car when they met. But she wasn't ever really in love with him . . . never mind. I am, as they say, getting ahead of myself.

In my mother's journal from the year before we brought her to California, there was a single entry:

> *Notes, April 18—Tom's birthday, far away in the Golden West. And again, I repeat my cry—if only the U.S.A. weren't so damned BIG!!! No easy visit with Tom or Ellie—$1000s for plane fare—@$/#**?!!& This written as I await André and Liz and the Murphys for dinner. Loneliness is the vicious symptom. Still smoking cigarettes—my only companions. Still too many martinis before supper—one is enough—three is dangerous—And am sick of my seasick stomach—STOP— ENOUGH—What causes this??*

Almost a decade after Mike's death, the tall old gray house was saturated with melancholy. It just about oozed from the walls. My mother had done pretty well in the first few years. She'd come out of her crushing grief enough to take a job as curator of the local historical museum. Her friends were fantastic. They took her out, invited her to parties, came to parties at her house. And they didn't just do it at the beginning and then drift away. If only every widowed person could be surrounded as she was by attentive, loyal friends, ranging in age from their twenties to their eighties, some of whom my mother had known since long before Mike. A few men—some of them suitors from the distant past— tried to court my mother, but they might as well have tried to woo the moon out of the sky. They were up against the memory of Mike, an impossible act to follow, and she would have none of it. When she speaks of her loneliness in her journal, it's not the classic widow's loneliness, the days and nights in front of the television, the silent telephone. Hardly. It's specific: It's loneliness for *Mike*.

When I tell people who never knew Mike what a great guy he was, and how my mother never got over his death, and how no man could ever take his place, they sometimes say that probably she romanticized him in her memory. But she didn't. He really was that great. It happens sometimes, a fluke of nature, the same way someone's born every once in a while who's evil, vile and rotten through and through.

He was kind, loving, compassionate, funny, brilliant, wise, generous and sweet. He was hardworking, prolific, responsible, reliable, honest, a passionate environmentalist with a huge social conscience. He was sunny, cheerful and optimistic. He loved to cook, was really good at it, and cleaned up the kitchen afterward. He sang and played the guitar. He did the laundry. He was a fine dancer. He was a fantastic listener. He was utterly faithful, cuddly and loads of fun. He and my mother were always cracking jokes, laughing helplessly. If only he'd had a serious defect or two, a bad habit or a dark dirty secret, even a small one. But he didn't. As far as I could see, he was virtually a man without fault. He did, however, have a fatal physical flaw. He was born with it, and it was what eventually killed him before his time.

For such a man to die seemed like a malicious blow from the universe. That's how my mother took it. She wasn't just heartbroken—she was furious. People found out quickly that they'd better put a lid on trying to offer spiritual comfort, unless they wanted to draw back the proverbial bloody stump. That kind of talk only cranked up her rage. "Mike's looking down on you and laughing," said one well-meaning person, "because he knows you'll be together again some day." "Baloney," my mother snapped. Or the woman who obviously didn't know her very well, whose ears are probably still smarting: "It's God's will," she said. This was in some public place—the post office, the food store, right after Mike's death. My mother whirled and struck like a snake.

"Then God is a murderer," she spat.

My mother's anger had always been dangerous and colorful, in the tradition of smart people with quick tongues. She could slice and dice an opponent with the best of them. I remember being a little kid watching her chew out a cab driver in Manhattan after he'd tried to overcharge her. She ended a withering blast of words with "You *jerk!*" and slammed the door shut in the guy's face while he sat there speechless. A few years after Mike's death, her temper grown perilously short, she scared off a young out-of-town couple who'd challenged her when her car door touched theirs in the parking lot in front of the food store. The encounter ended with them locking their doors and peeling out in a big hurry.

My mother always thought that since she was so much older than Mike she'd die first. But she has Methuselah genes on both sides of her family, and might have outlived him even if he hadn't died young. It was her sheer physical toughness that kept her shattered heart beating and her arms and legs moving despite grief that might have killed someone else.

So, with time and a little help from her friends, she rallied. For a good while. She even wrote another book, a lively history of the town's local Lake Waramaug (Indian chiefs, bootleggers, whorehouses, renegades, aristocrats, violinmakers, and so forth). Nobody could write history like my mother. As a fiction writer, she had a powerful gift for character development. When she wrote about real people from another time, she used that same gift, sniffing out the most bizarre and fascinating aspects of their adventures and misadventures like a detective. My mother and Mike coauthored *On the Road with John James Audubon,* considered one of the definitive works on the great artist-naturalist. They traced Audubon's travels all over the country, from the Florida Keys to Labrador to the Mississippi, and kept diaries and notes as they went. For a year and a half they camped and cooked over fires and had a ball. My mother said it was the absolute best time of both their lives. There are three voices in the book—Audubon's, Mike's, and my mother's. It's a superb triple counterpoint: Audubon the flamboyant artist and explorer, writing in his diary in the early 1800s when the continent was a shaggy wilderness, and then, more than a century and a half later, Mike the environmentalist and journalist and my mother the narrative historian and keen social observer, in all the places Audubon visited, some of which had scarcely changed and others of which were unrecognizable. The personalities of Audubon, his long-suffering wife, the entrepreneurs and scalawags Audubon encountered in his travels and those my mother and Mike encountered in theirs come to vivid life under my mother's pen.

She and the Waramaug project were a perfect match: This had been her territory since childhood. For the two years she worked on the book she was passionately occupied—racing around the lake taking pictures, interviewing old-timers, searching through diaries, letters and newspaper archives all the way back to the 1700s. At home, drafts and photos and papers covered every surface in the kitchen and dining room and her ancient black upright manual typewriter shook the house. Just like the old days.

The book turned out to be a little gem, its sales far surpassing the expectations of the preservation committee that commissioned her for the job. Word got out, and people who didn't know Lake Waramaug from Lake Wobegon were snapping it up from the shelves of the bookstore.

Yes. She came back for a while, heroically. But Mike was everywhere in the house long after he was gone. The place was riddled with snares and booby traps. In the basement, their camping gear from the Audubon travels languished, including cooking utensils and spices, as if maybe my mother and Mike might jump in the car and take off on an adventure at any moment. Moldering bags of flour, remnants of his bread-baking, sat in a barrel in the kitchen four and five years after his death. On the wall by the phone, numbers in his handwriting. He could have come back to life at any time and walked into his study and sat right back down at his computer and gone to work. My mother lifted a cushion off a chair about seven years after he died, found his pocketknife and burst into tears. Soon after that, she discovered two loaves of his bread in the bottom of the deep freeze in the basement. Whenever I called her on the phone, I could always hear the strain of grief in her voice when she said hello. It never eased the way everyone said it would. It just got worse.

My brother, Tom, and I had thought she should leave the house as soon as she could after Mike's death, that a change of scenery was desperately needed. She'd been alone and lonely in that house before—after Durant and pre-Mike. Then Mike was in her life for twenty-three years. Now, incredibly, she was alone in that house again. Sometimes she agreed that she should leave, sometimes she didn't. She said it was true that there were doleful memories in abundance, but that there were happy memories, too. In any case, she'd been there since 1955. It was a three-story house packed from attic to basement. The prospect of emptying the place and moving was huge, daunting, and even though she herself eventually decided it was time to go and started tackling closets and drawers and boxes, an actual move kept getting put off another year, and another and another.

She was willing to leave that house, but she didn't want to leave the town. Not yet. She wanted to find another place there, maybe a condo. She wanted to stay for as long as she could in the green hills of Connecticut, with her friends, the people who had known Mike. She always said that: I want to be around the people who knew Mike. She wanted to stay where her life was. Until she got too old, she always said.

The Waramaug book turned out to be her last hurrah. She finished it in 1996, but not without a struggle in the home stretch. In retrospect, we see that the beast already had its first tentative hooks in her.

A few years ago, my mother called me in California to tell me she'd won a Ford Taurus in a sweepstakes. She said her plan was to take the cash value instead and give half the money to me and half to my brother. I got all excited. My mother's always been generous, always ready to share, never any strings. Always on our side.

There was no Ford Taurus, though. My mother, the laser-eyed editor and incomparable wordsmith, had been fooled by the tricky language on the "award" notice.

Soon after, Tom, who lives in Colorado, got a call from my mother's bank. "This might be none of our business," they said, "but we thought you should know: Your mother has taken out two cashier's checks recently, one last week for five grand, and just today, another for three, both made out to the same party."

Everyone knows each other in her little town. Tommy called the local post office, reaching them a few minutes before the day's mail went out. The postmaster did what could have cost him his job—fished through the bin and found the envelope with my mother's name and return address on it. It was going to a P.O. box in Montreal. Inside was the check for three thousand dollars.

My brother talked to my mother. Some really nice woman had called her from Canada, told her she'd won fifty thousand dollars in a sweepstakes. All she had to do was pay the taxes on it first. With cashier's checks. There was a time when my mother, one of the sharpest people I've ever known, would have eaten such flim-flam artists for lunch and picked her teeth with their bones.

The first check, the one for five grand, was lost forever. She cried and berated herself. She said she was going to divide the fifty thousand between the three of us.

"It's not the money, Mom," my brother said to her gently, kindly. "And that was a wonderful impulse. But something's seriously wrong here. Do you remember when I was there a few months ago, and I took the phone out of your hand because you were starting to give some total stranger your checking account number?"

"No," she said. "I don't remember."

There had been other portents in the last year or so. I'd shoved them aside. My mother's invincibility was a cornerstone of my life. There had been a sad little episode that we reconstructed from bits and pieces: She'd driven to Maine to visit an old friend (who was slipping himself— he'd recently passed through town writing bad checks), got mixed up asking directions at a toll booth, got mad, tried to back up, rammed the car behind her. And now her friends were calling Tommy and me, telling us things weren't right at all, that she was confused, bursting into tears in public, forgetting the way to people's houses where she'd been going for decades, denting up her car, repeating questions five times during a phone conversation, then calling up and asking the same questions again, drinking too much, sliding back into obsessively mourning Mike, selling valuable things in her house to crooks, bouncing from doctor to doctor with a mysterious chronic stomach upset that seemed to have no physical cause. The only thing that settled her stomach, she told us, was her evening vodka martini.

My brother hadn't shoved anything aside, though. He was adamant. She's only going to get worse, he said. We can't just sit and wait for disaster. We have to preempt it. We have to get her out. Now. One more winter alone there and something really bad will happen.

I would never have had the spine to make such a decision, but he did. It looks to me like Alzheimer's, he said.

Alzheimer's?

He may as well have suggested elephantiasis. Not possible, I said. Not her. All our ancient relatives kept their marbles right up to the end. She's just—I don't know, depressed or something. It must be all the prescription drugs she's taking. For her chronic upset stomach, for insomnia, for depression. But it couldn't be . . . Alzheimer's.

That might have been the first time I ever spoke the word in some context other than cracking jokes about public figures.

But then I remembered another small, uneasy moment I'd relegated to some locked trunk in a corner of my mind, and experienced a nasty and prescient little squirt of adrenaline recollecting it: My mother, on a recent visit to California, standing in front of my house looking at my car, a peculiar baffled, scared expression around her eyes.

Where's *my* car? she said.

Her car, of course, was nearly three thousand miles away, in Connecticut.

CHAPTER TWO

The Serpent's Tooth

My brother and I share a malaise. We call it Connecticut Melancholia. There are specific sounds that we sometimes imitate over the telephone to each other when we want to evoke it: katydids, for instance. Any New Englander will know what I'm talking about here. The katydids start up in late summer, in the evening. At first you just hear a stray one here and there. It always seems too early. It's only August, goddamnit! Within a week or so, the night fairly vibrates with their raspy three-syllable one-note song, which they make with their hind legs. You might even find a katydid once in a while. They're astonishing bugs, big and lusciously, delicately green with intricate veined transparent wings. The old timers say the advent of the katydids means six weeks until the first frost. It awakens in me a primal sadness: Summer's dying. Here comes fall, then winter. Back-to-school, back-to-school, back-to-school, say the katydids. And that first frost shuts the katydids up decisively. Overnight, they're silenced.

When my brother and I really want to lay the Connecticut Melancholia on thick for one another, we also imitate church bells, the cawing of crows and the incomparably desolate (to us) sound of tires on the wet road going by my mother's house.

We're both afflicted. I had a mild case of it long before Mike died. It was always stronger for my brother. We each left Connecticut early, before either of us was twenty years old. For him, the antidote was the big sky and vastness of the Colorado Rockies. For me, it was also Colorado for a while and then California. But I used to enjoy long visits in the golden days when Mike was there. We had good times. I'd stay for a while, then, satisfied, head back out west. Even my brother liked an occasional visit.

In the years since Mike's death the melancholia grew so that it was almost unbearable for us to be in Connecticut at all, and the house made us so sad we could hardly stand to walk through the door. And of course, it was after Mike's death that my mother wanted us there the most. When she asked when we were coming to visit, there was always a little ragged edge to the question, a plea that she couldn't suppress. If we had to go, spring was by far the least melancholy time of year. Next was summer, as long as there was no risk of late-August katydids. Fall? Beautiful, but dangerous. Late fall, when the leaves are mostly brown and about to forsake the trees entirely and that chill foreboding is in the air? Uh-uh. Winter? Naked trees against gray skies? Stone walls in the snowy woods like tombstones? Forget it.

When Tommy or I visited her in Connecticut after Mike was gone, we could never stay as long as she wanted us to. A couple of weeks was the most I could manage; even that was too long for my brother. That old melancholia would set its teeth in us no matter what the season and we'd get antsy and anxious to go. And she'd know it. And then there she'd be, a forlorn figure standing there at the bus stop in Southbury waving good-bye. It was too sad. And she never failed to tell us, half-jokingly for a while and then maybe only one-third jokingly and then one-tenth, that she wished we'd move home.

It was getting a little too real. Both of us had an uneasy lurking vision of the town somehow reclaiming us, that no matter how far we went or for how long, we'd end up back there. It's hard to explain the melancholia. When we tell people about it, they always say: But the town and the countryside are so beautiful! And there are so many extraordinary characters living there, such an amazing sociological mix! All that is true, and it's all part of the problem. The place is powerfully seductive. But for us, it's also cramped, confining, decaying, too redolent with ancient smells and sounds. Both of us know that if we ever stayed for any length of time, whatever shreds of youth we still have would be sucked right out of us. Like a reverse Shangri-La.

My brother has a theory: He says the Connecticut malaise has its origins in the Tim Durant years. That the feeling is the leftover sorrow of missing our mother acutely because Durant was always taking her away somewhere. He could be right. It could all be Durant's fault. His fault that we both went and lived thousands of miles from home, his fault that forty years after he left we had to go and rip my mother out of the place she loved because we couldn't go live there. And of course, my mother chose him, over a crowd of suitors.

Christ, the way we sow the seeds of our destinies . . .

I had for years entertained a fond but hazy vision of my mother eventually moving out to California to live near me. We'd have fun. We'd be together. Especially with Mike gone, I was always sorry about the vast continent between us and all the time that went by without the two of us seeing each other. I could give her so much more of my time and attention if I didn't have to go to Connecticut to do it. And she always said that eventually—eventually—she'd like to move west.

The moment of bringing her to California arrived rudely, at the absolute worst possible time. I was anything but ready. The vicissitudes of the publishing world had conspired to put me in a situation where I had about six months to write most of a long-overdue manuscript. Just when I should have been buckling down to what would have been, even under the best of circumstances, a gruelingly concentrated push to finish, I—the world's most terrified flier, my terror compounded tenfold by terror of what I would be doing when I landed—was getting on a plane to the East Coast, without a prayer of getting any writing done for what I thought would be weeks and weeks. Ah. If only it had been mere weeks and weeks . . .

And it was early autumn, mid-September. The katydids were in full voice the night we arrived.

She flung her arms around us at the door just as she did whenever we came to visit. I'd been bringing Mitch, my mate, to Connecticut for

years by then. We always slept down in Mike's study on the first floor.
There's a door there that opens onto the back terrace; if it was summer,
fall or spring, which it always was because I couldn't stand to be there
in the winter, we'd open it wide and let the night air waft over us, pro-
ducing olfactory synesthesia of the Third Kind. The house looks out
over a river valley. We'd lie there and listen to the water and the night
sounds and smell the rich moist East Coast aromas of whatever season
it was, so different from California smells. The visits were like gold to
my mother. She'd have little parties for us. We talked and drank and had
fun. Mitch was charming and gallant with her. She adored him.

Fate, whatever your definition of it or your beliefs about its
mechanics, is indeed a mysterious thing. Mitch never met Mike, but
years ago, in 1978, before he knew me or my mother, he'd saved an issue
of *Harper's* magazine because of the important cover story, "Oil and
Water." It was about the environmental effect of oil spills, a subject near
and dear to him. It was by Michael Harwood. He has that magazine to
this day. Now here he was, sleeping in the very room where the piece
had been written, the artifacts of the deceased author all around him,
including the typewriter it was written on. I picture Mitch holding that
Harper's in his hands twenty years before, in California, looking at the
cover, at the name Michael Harwood. Little could he have imagined
that this man's death would someday almost turn his life inside out.

Yes, she'd flung her arms around us at the door, as if this were going
to be a fun visit. My gizzard was in my mouth. I'm not good at betrayal, and no matter how we sliced it, the job we were there to do was
going to involve betrayal. The reasons were all in place, and they were
sound, and we had talked about it and talked about it with her, all summer long, but of course by the time it's necessary to move a person out
of her home because she can't take care of herself anymore it's already
too late for good sound reasons to make any sense to her. And she was
still so much like her old self most of the time. If it had been just me,
who caves in at the smallest yelp of pain from someone I love, especially from my mother, I would probably have pretended everything was
fine and visited for a while and maybe had a few pleading and ineffec-
tual conversations, and then I would have gone home to California and

left her in her house for another winter. And I don't know what would
have happened. But I was impaled by doubt. I waffled and agonized. Is
this really necessary? Do we really have to do this? Aren't we seriously
jumping the gun here? Is she really that bad?

The trust officer who managed the small estate left to my mother
by Mike's life insurance and savings, and who was personally fond of
her, was not troubled by any doubts. He was downright forceful. I've
seen it so many times in my line of work, he said. So many times. Old
people ignored by their offspring, left alone in their houses, losing their
memories and their competence, getting ripped off and abused by
opportunists, drinking, setting themselves on fire, crashing their cars. If
something happens to your mother, he said, and you two are thousands
of miles away, and she gets committed to a hospital and becomes a ward
of the state, then you will have the devil's own time, legally and finan-
cially, extricating her from the system. Don't let it happen. Don't wait
until it's too late.

And there was her stomach. A few years before, little packets of over-
the-counter antacids started to appear: around her house, in the medicine cabinet, on the dashboard of her car, in the pockets of her pants.
Now there were bottles of prescription medicines from three and four
different gastroenterologists, overlapping appointments scrawled on her
calendar. She'd gone to the Yale-New Haven Hospital and the Sharon
Hospital for tests. No one could find anything wrong. The S.O.S. calls
from her friends to my brother and me had included stories of my
mother ricocheting from one doctor to another, mixing up appointments, forgetting which doctors she'd been to, pestering some of them
after they'd exhausted every avenue so that some of them were refusing
to see her anymore. I called one whose name I found on five or six of
the dozens of prescription bottles in the kitchen, bedroom, bathroom.

"You realize that your mother is suffering from dementia, don't
you?" said the voice on the other end of the line, without sympathy.

"Uh, yes," I said. *Jesus. What a weird horrible ugly word.*

"Your mother got hold of my home number. She called me there
four times in one day. My wife was very upset."

"I apologize. It won't happen again."

"I'm glad to hear that."

"It's just that her stomach is driving her crazy. She's desperate for help. Do you have any idea at all what's wrong?"

"Probably irritable bowel syndrome."

"Ah. Hmm. Irritable bowel syndrome. Well, so, what's the treatment?"

"There is no treatment."

I was looking out over the heartbreakingly beautiful view from the back of the house. The leaves were just starting to turn. It was plain that this doctor's stomach wasn't bothering him the least little bit. No treatment? Screw you, I thought. I apologized again for my mother's importunity and hung up.

Just about every day now, the Stomach Monster reared its head. Usually in the early afternoon, right after lunch. She described it as nausea, like morning sickness or seasickness, sometimes punctuated by shooting pains and a dizzy, shaky feeling. She'd lie on the couch as if she'd been bonked with a two-by-four. My mother had never been sickly. She'd had little patience with people who constantly complained about their physical problems. And now here she was, plagued by a mystery malady, and losing her judgment and the ability to systematically follow through with a course of treatment or a change of diet. The only thing that helped was her evening vodka martini. She'd have one, and then she'd have another . . . and sometimes another.

The stomach grief had taken a major turn for the worse since I'd last seen her, in May. Witnessing it up close now, it seemed to me to be her most urgent problem. The daily misery and distress aggravated her confusion and depression, drove her to desperate actions and excessive drink. It stood in the way of her just plain feeling good, the first logical step, I thought, toward improving her life. And it was obvious that unless someone took charge of running the cause of this thing to earth, and conscientiously and consistently experimenting and applying treatments because she was no longer capable of any of this herself, everything would spiral inevitably downward. We could not leave her alone any longer.

So, with a quaking heart, I screwed my feeble resolve to the sticking point. Fortunately, no one was looking to me to provide cohesion and impetus. My brother was the backbone of this operation. My mother had voluntarily made him her conservator within the past year, after her blunders with the Canadian crooks, and he was taking the responsibility seriously. If saving her from an ignominious decline and possible down-the-road disaster meant causing some pain now, then he was willing to do it. He's worked as a ski-patrol Emergency Medical Technician in Colorado, so he's trained at handling hairy life-and-death situations in a businesslike way. Unlike me. I'd heard of "tough love," but I'd always associated it with juvenile delinquents and such. Tough? Love? Never did I dream that I'd have to practice this oxymoronic concept on my mother.

We got down to it quickly. Things went amazingly well. She agreed that it was time to get out, that she couldn't possibly do it by herself, and that we should get started. She seemed almost eager. My guts began to settle into their normal arrangement. We spent a day walking through the entire house with her while she chose what she wanted to keep and what she was willing to let go. She was decisive and sensible, keeping just a few pieces for sentimental reasons. We conscientiously double-checked with her over each item. "Are you sure?" "I'm sure," she said. We arranged for a couple of auctioneers to collect the things she was willing to part with.

As they loaded up their truck with furniture, dishes, her brass bed, her silver, breaking the set after a forty-three-year run, I wanted to go hide. It was a moment I'd been seriously dreading. I expected a scene. But she watched calmly. A little too calmly, now that I think about it.

That evening after dinner, Mitch was resting and my brother and I sat at the dining room table with her. Tommy and I were quietly elated. The worst was over. We were telling her about the groovy little apartment we'd found for her in my seaside town in northern California. A view of the ocean. Cozy, gorgeous, a block away from me. We'd send out the things she'd kept, make the apartment welcoming and cozy. Her trusty old manual typewriter would be waiting for her. She could write her memoirs. Be near me. A new life, we said. She listened, looking pleased. Much had been accomplished that day. A lot of furniture was gone, but we'd rearranged things so that the house was still comfortable and homey.

"Oh, by the way," she said, lighting a cigarette, "I've decided to put this move off until spring."

"Uh ... Mom," said my brother, "you can't. We talked about this. It's all we've been talking about. It's why we're here right now. It's ... "

"I WON'T GO!!" she shrieked, jolting us out of our skins. She leapt from her chair and ran into the other room. I jumped up and ran after her. She cowered on the sofa, weeping, shaking, her hands over her face. I approached, put my arms around her, tried to soothe her, but she slithered out of my grasp and ran back into the other room. "NO!" she shouted, whacking the table with the flat of her hand, plates and forks and glasses clattering. I went toward her again, supplicating. She dodged behind the chairs. "NO, NO, NO!" Could it get any worse? We, her hulking full-grown spawn, retro-children quaking at her thunder, chasing her around the room.

It took time and a lot of talking, but we did manage to calm her, reassure her, remind her what we were doing and why, though by then it was sounding more than a little hollow and tinny to my own ears. Exhausted, we all went to bed.

My mother's footsteps had always been eloquent, especially in that house. The house is on a hillside that slopes down from a road, so when you walk in the front door, which faces the road, you are on the second floor. The kitchen is on that floor now. My mother's study and a couple of bedrooms, including hers, were on the third floor. Mike's study and what had been the kitchen back in the old days when my brother and I were kids is on the first floor. The house, old and made of wood, resonates like a drum.

She was an afternoon napper, and woe to anyone who woke her up. Sound traveled easily up the old radiator pipes, so if we were fooling around on the first floor it was possible to disturb her on the third. And she moved fast: We'd hear running footsteps, and scatter. Or later, when we were teenagers, partying downstairs late at night with friends, and heard *boom-boom-boom-boom-boom!* on the top floor and heading down the stairs, we'd crowd out the back door like slapstick comedians in a silent film. Her wrath had nothing to do with us smoking dope and drinking beer and staying up all night. She didn't give a damn about that. "I was SLEEPING!" she'd yell.

I overheard a conversation between her and Durant once, on the second floor. I must have been about eight. They didn't know I'd come up the stairs and was in the next room. There were scuffles and whispers. She was crying, her voice anguished but low so my brother and I wouldn't hear. "You don't want me. You don't *need* me!" she said, and ran up the stairs—*boom-boom-boom-boom-boom!*—to the bedroom.

Now, on the terrible night that she'd run away from us, I lay awake in the wee hours on the floor of Mike's study. I listened to my mother's agitated footsteps overhead, up and down the stairs, up and down, pacing, pacing, pacing. I tried to put myself in her mind, but I couldn't. She was on another planet.

The house looked strange, of course. Furniture and art and books I'd been seeing for forty years were gone. There were peculiar blank spaces. The house was becoming a visible metaphor of my mother's mind.

A couple of rooms stayed untouched. The upstairs storage room, the kitchen, and her study. I wanted badly to get into that study. Somewhere in the geological layers were my mother's Lost Works. I desperately wanted to get my hands on them. I read and re-read her novels every couple of years, especially the first one. But these lost things I hadn't seen for ages.

There was, for instance, a hilarious series of letters she'd written to Richard Nixon in the seventies, in the deadpan voice of a not-too-literate housewife protesting, say, the waste of gasoline to fly all those "aeroplanes" in military airshows when in her day "the Drum and Bugle Corps marched for free." The letters were always written by hand in a purposely laborious cursive script and signed "Yours in the Flag, Mrs. Mary Harwood." They got passed around among her literati friends and were gleefully called the "Yours in the Flag" letters. The only responses she got from the White House were form letters of the "Thank you for your interest" type.

And there were some short stories—eerie little *Outer Limits*-like gems, never published, buried (I hoped) deep in her files. There was one called "The Soul of Mrs. Gurney" that I really, really wanted to find. It was about a man and wife, married forever, harnessed together like two mules, mired in habit and routine. It ended with the usually docile submissive husband using an arcane bit of voodoo he gleans from an obscure little book to sever his wife's soul from her body while she's dreaming. And there was another story, called "The Hunting Knife," a dark tale of an older woman's flirtation with a teenage boy who has criminal tendencies. I hadn't seen these stories since before I was a teenager, but their quality was obvious to me even then. And there was the third novel, never finished, about hobo kids during the Depression, started in the seventies but abandoned when the Audubon project came along.

There was another item I was particularly keen to find, and I did. It was on the top shelf of the closet in the guest room on the third floor: a big glossy black-and-white photograph, with "Irish News Agency, 1954" stamped on the back. It was the original of John Huston kissing my mother at her wedding to Durant. Ha! I was elated. I'd thought it was lost forever, and now here it was in my hands. Tomorrow I'd make copies so I could flash it around to my friends back home. How many of them had pictures of their mothers being kissed by John Huston? I'd always liked bragging about my mother. I could do some serious showing off with this picture.

A few hours later, the picture had vanished from where I left it atop the bureau. I looked everywhere, including my mother's study, packed with books and papers. I asked her if she had moved it. Did you hide it? Put it in a book or something? Think hard, I begged. I really wanted that picture.

But she couldn't remember—either whether she had moved it, or if she had, where she might have put it. It was just gone. I eyed her crammed study. It's somewhere in there, I thought. It could be in a thousand different places in there, but that's where it is.

One day soon after the auctioneers had taken away the furniture, my brother and I made a foray into her study, to try to at least start organizing the stacks and piles and boxes. She stopped us. "No," she said. "I'll do this myself." I could hardly blame her. By then it was obvious what her son and daughter, whom she loved unconditionally, had become: a marauding army. She still loved us, though, even after all of this. I deferred to her, though I was dreadfully worried that she'd throw things out that I wanted to find—like her stories.

A few days before it was time for us to leave, an old friend stepped in gallantly to help. Phil, a theatre pal from decades back, came up from New York to stay for a while so that when we left she wouldn't be abruptly and echoingly alone in her strangely half-empty house. He'd go back to New York and come up again toward the end of October to spend the final week with her. He'd help her pack, make sure she stuck to the plan. Then Mike's best buddy, Dave, would escort her and her cat, Polly, out on the airplane.

Mitch and I would go out to California and get everything ready. We'd make her happy. No more dinners alone, lots of loving attention, vitamins, acupuncturists. I'd get right to work on the stomach problem. I'd restore her faltering memory. Give her a new life.

We spent October fixing up her apartment in California. The place looked exquisite. I began to experience a sort of forgetfulness myself. Here were her books and pictures. Here was a nice long table with her typewriter on it. Here was a view of the ocean. My mother was coming. My fun wonderful brilliant mother. There'd be jolly dinners. Parties. She'd make friends.

She arrived on schedule at the end of October.

On the ride home from the airport with her and Dave and the cat, we told her we were all going to go to her wonderful apartment. She started crying. "Apartment? What apartment? I thought I was going to be living with you," she said. Something akin to panic started to push open a door in my head, but I shoved it closed.

We soothed her and reassured her. She seemed to like the apartment. When I put her to bed that night, she said: "You want me. You really want me." "Of course I do," I said, hearing that hollow tinny sound again.

She got a new life, all right, and so did we.

CHAPTER THREE

The Undead

Northern California winters are wet and raw. It rains and rains and rains. Storms blow in from thousands of miles out in the Pacific and pound the remote coastline where we live, three hours north of San Francisco. High winds and crashing trees snuff the power for days at a time. That November brought winter howling in along with my mother. She arrived on Halloween night.

In Anne Rice's *Interview with the Vampire,* we are given a vivid taste of the breaking-in process by which a mortal becomes a vampire: One's body is agonizingly, bewilderingly, gradually but surely cleansed of all life until one is completely . . . undead.

Those first couple of months were a similar breaking-in for us. Mitch and I were cleansed not only of our former lives but of delusions. Though we were still like the proverbial blind men feeling an elephant in the dark, we started to get a good idea of the size and shape of the beast called Alzheimer's.

I saw a picture recently of a brain diseased by Alzheimer's. It had been sliced horizontally, and the perspective was from above, as if you were looking down on a tree stump. Like a tree stump, there were concentric rings—but the rings were of nothingness, as if the disease eats the brain according to its own biologically programmed pattern, the destruction random as it tunnels through the various sections where the different functions reside. The disease isn't particular. To it, brain tissue is brain tissue, all of it equally tasty.

If I'd seen that picture back when I was setting out to rescue my mother, would I still have done what I did? I don't know. I do know that I was ignorant. Profoundly, prodigiously ignorant.

They used to talk about aluminum pots and pans maybe causing Alzheimer's. Then, for a while, they were talking about a possible connection to Mad Cow disease. You hear something new every day. The inflammation theory, which is not at all inconsistent with the latter, makes sense—there's an apparent correlation between regular ibuprofin use and a lower risk of Alzheimer's. Virus? Heredity? Environment? A combination of the three? They don't know for sure yet, but what's known is this: The prognosis is progressive, irreversible memory loss, delusions and disorientation until you don't recognize your children, your husband, your wife—the process more gradual in some people than in others—and eventually you forget to eat, swallow, breathe.

In the same way that all cancer is illness but not all illness is cancer, all Alzheimer's is dementia but not all dementia is Alzheimer's. There are different causes of dementia: Heavy alcohol use can do it. So can certain nutritional deficiencies, mini-strokes, and so forth. Whatever the cause, the different types of dementia tend to resemble each other. It is, after all, the same organ, the brain, that's breaking down. When I took on my mother's illness, a definitive diagnosis of Alzheimer's could only be made post mortem. Since then, I've heard about weird, Island-of-Dr.-Moreau-type diagnostic procedures, like drilling a hole in the skull and taking a core sample of brain matter, or injecting a protein dye into the head and "reading" it somehow. Again, if I'd known about those tests back then, would I have put her through them? They sound ghastly, nightmarishly primitive, an insult to her body and soul. Such questions, though, are thoroughly moot. We did what we did, and it's way too late now to look back. What I did know was that the vast majority of dementia cases are indeed Alzheimer's, so the likelihood was high that this was what she had. If it wasn't Alzheimer's, I'd find out what it was and fix it. No matter what, though, I was not ready to consign my

mother to the bone heap. Even if it was Alzheimer's, I'd beat it. And I'd
make her happy.

I mentioned ignorance. Did I mention hubris?

Stability and predictability in daily routine are what the sages prescribe
for people with Alzheimer's or any variety of dementia. They are also
fonts of wise words for the caregivers: Take care of yourself, they all say.
Give yourself a break. Be sure to set aside time to do the things you
enjoy. Get plenty of rest. Pamper yourself. Enlist the help of friends and
relatives to assist with your "Loved One." Take time out for yourself,
they chant. Time out for yourself. I'll let you in on a secret: There is no
time out, not even when you are sound asleep, if the person is in fact a
loved one AND money is scarce as rain in the Sahara. That's the one
they never mention when they're telling you to get plenty of help and
plenty of rest, the one thing without which there will be no help and
no rest: For God's sake, have plenty of money.

If the "help" books discuss the subject at all, they're demure and ret-
icent. But I'm going to risk being indelicate and indecorous. I'm going
to discuss it. I'm going to be crass and shout it at the top of my lungs.
There's a saying we've all heard: *The rich are different from you and me.* I
can think of few life situations that will teach you the true meaning of
this little string of words better than trying to take care of someone with
Alzheimer's and having to do it all yourself. The heartbreak, chaos and
destruction that come with the disease will be exacerbated and magnified in direct proportion to how broke you are. This is simply the truth.
Without the protection of money, the strain starts to kill you right away.

Money. It can't buy back a person's mind, that's for sure, but it can
absolutely help you save your own. My mother arrived with some
monthly money. Mitch and I are both writers, a polite term for "occasional pauper." In other words, sometimes we had to do other things for
income. I was under contract to write a novel set in eighth-century
China; indentured, I should say, the advance by then a dim memory. The
time when Mitch would have been doing other things for money to
support the household had to go to my mother's care and attention. We
in our perfect naiveté and our cockeyed optimism had not anticipated

just how much care and attention that would be. What this equation meant was that we became dependent on her modest money almost immediately, not counting whatever cash came from work Mitch was able to squeeze in.

The sages—advice books, help hotlines and such—presume a certain level of solid middle-class fiscal security, and take it from there. They don't tell you what to do if your agent is too busy jet-setting around with movie stars and billionaires to communicate with your overseas publisher to find out that the publishers moved their offices from one city in Germany to another and lost your manuscript, and that the original editor who commissioned the work has quit and the new editor wants a revised storyline, and now you have to start all over, advance money spent, with an insanely foreshortened deadline and your brokenhearted, uprooted, bewildered, grieving Alzheimered mother needing you twenty-four hours a day. Nope; they don't have much to say about that. Take a bubble bath. Go to the movies. Be sure to get plenty of rest.

Lack of money, as some of us know, produces its own special anxiety, and so there was an abundance of that along with exotic new strains of anxiety I'd not been exposed to before. Their juices bathed my nervous system every day along with a heaping helping of good old-fashioned guilt. Guilt over dragging my mother away from her home, guilt over what I was inflicting on Mitch. He'd been a single father, had raised three children from diapers to adulthood. He'd more than earned his freedom, and now, because of me, he was in a domestic trap again. This is not fair, I thought. This is not what he signed on for. We weren't even officially married; he was under no obligation to stay.

"I'll do this," he said at the beginning, "but I can't promise I'll always be nice."

I knew he would not quit or walk away. The fact that he'd raised children meant he was way better prepared for what we'd taken on than I, who'd assiduously avoided parenthood because I never wanted the responsibility. It was both reassuring and alarming to know he was in it for the duration. The whites of his eyes were showing after only a week or so of my mother's presence, and we were looking at infinity.

And it wasn't as if she had forced herself on us. She'd cried and screamed, run away from us. She didn't want to be here, but we'd brought her, and it was my responsibility to make her happy. What have we done? whispered the voice of doom and dread when my eyes popped open at dawn shortly after her arrival. *What have we done?*

My mother and I, like a lot of mothers and daughters, share particular bonds. One of our strongest is a little—um—different from the usual.

About ten years ago, on my birthday, an elderly lady friend of mine here in California threw me a small party. The other guests were mostly older people, too, in their seventies and eighties, pals of hers who were regulars at her frequent tea parties. A wrapped gift from my mother had arrived in the mail a few days before. It felt like a big book. I took it along, still wrapped, to the birthday tea party so I could open it there along with the other little gifts I'd be getting.

After cake and tea, funny hat on my head, I unwrapped presents, saving my mother's for last. While everyone watched, I pulled off the paper. I was right; it was a big book. Red, with large black letters: *Hunting Humans—An Encyclopedia of Modern Serial Killers*. The guests were a worldly group, so they weren't overly shocked. I passed the book around and they all looked at it. But I know they thought it a bit . . . curious that a mother would give such a birthday gift to her daughter. It wasn't curious to me. I was thrilled.

About ten years before that, when I was on a visit to Connecticut, my mother and I drove a fair distance to the shop of a rare book dealer, where we bought a circa 1890s tome called *Anomalies and Curiosities of Medicine*. This book had pictures. Lots of pictures. On the ride back, my mother and I, screaming and laughing, swerved all over the road looking at the book.

I have on my shelf another book she gave me, called *Wisconsin Death Trip,* a superb collection of haunting photographs and copy from a defunct newspaper in a Wisconsin town around the turn of the last century. I have a dozen old medical and pathology books full of strange pictures. I have books on forensics and true crime. Half of these were presents from my mother. I once gave her a nineteenth-century obstetrics book that would cause a steep decline in birth rates if enough women saw it.

What we share is a taste for the *noir,* an interest in the macabre which, a family friend once observed, was incipient in my grandmother, well-developed in my mother and fully realized in me. Some people understand it, some don't. It has to do with a certain literal-mindedness and a touch of nihilism—a fascination with, and a reaction to, the reality of entropy and death. There's an aesthetic dimension to it as well. It can serve, be a rich source of creative inspiration. It's a proclivity I'm grateful to have.

There is a flip side, though: It can, if circumstances are just so, get out of its cage and keep you awake at night with lurid visions of decay and disaster. The voice of doom and dread.

But then there's crazy optimism, too—in my case, a partial leftover from an idealistic stage of my youth, but at the time of my mother's arrival born mostly of perfect ignorance and a reluctance to relinquish the notion that she was indestructible. Optimism and despair vied for ascendance. I clung to my hopeful visions like a castaway clutching a seat cushion. We took her to a good doctor, got her checked out completely. He put her on antidepressants. A psychologist tested her and diagnosed her with "probable" Alzheimer's. I did some research. I read about plaques and tangles in the brain, lipofuscin gumming up the neurotransmitters and such. I ordered special brain nutrients, not available stateside, over the Internet. Mitch actually made a trip down to Tijuana to get more.

And he made a significant discovery within a week of her arrival: She was putting away formidable amounts of vodka. He marked her bottle a couple of times, and found that during the night, after bedtime, not counting evening cocktails, the contents of the bottle dropped by a full two measuring cups. My mother weighs about 125 soaking wet. We saw the effect on her of a couple of martinis, and it was truly scary. As if she'd been punched in the head by Muhammed Ali. One night shortly after she arrived we went out to dinner and had drinks. During the dinner, she asked whether we were in Southbury or New Milford. These, of course, are towns in Connecticut. Afterward, we went to the all-night Safeway, and my mother stood there under the fluorescent lights with real terror on her face, and said, "I don't have the slightest idea where I am or why."

My mother had always been a controlled, moderate evening cocktail drinker. Never, ever when I was growing up did I see her even a little tipsy, and she was utterly disdainful of sloppy drunks. But nine years of desolation and now memory loss had done their insidious work. She still proclaimed that she never drank more than a couple of martinis a day, and only around dinnertime. It wasn't that she was lying or covering up. It was that she couldn't remember. We'd known for a couple of years that she was drinking more than she should, but none of us suspected just how much until Mitch marked her bottle.

Mitch's theory, the possibility that maybe her memory loss was booze-induced, seemed like a major revelation. God, we thought—maybe we can get my mother back just by sobering her up. And maybe sobering her up will fix everything else. Her stomach, for instance. She tippled during the day and in the wee hours to soothe her gastric distress, but her new doctor said that alcohol could act both as a temporary palliative and be the hidden culprit at the same time—and, he agreed, it could be the cause of her memory loss. A true vicious circle now a vicious downward spin. And maybe her feeling lousy and shaky was just a hangover!

So we got her off the hard stuff completely, gave her alcohol-less wine instead. We made a ceremony of it: ice cubes clinking cheerily and suggestively at the "cocktail hour." We knew it might take some time to see real results, but now we had something tangible to work with.

And every night, when I escorted her back to her apartment a block away, I laid out handfuls of vitamins, supplements, brain nutrients, herbal stomach soothers, her antidepressant, digestive enzymes . . . ah, yes. Our hopes were high.

Looking back, I can't even remember what that felt like. It was a gradual Invasion of the Body Snatchers. This person looked like my mother, dressed like my mother, sounded like my mother, but she was becoming everything that had been anathema to her: Intrusive. Complaining. Hypochondriacal.

And that thing that most of us would rather die than be, designated by Oscar Wilde as the only valid criterion by which one divides up the human race, the condition she would have dreaded most of all: Tedious.

The friends and good times I had envisioned did not materialize. Brain nutrients and abstinence were but one part of our attack. When she first arrived, I also worked hard to introduce her to people. I took her to singing groups, parties, meetings of the local Audubon Society. Tragic factors became quickly evident: When I did introduce her to someone, she forgot that person instantly. A long, fun dinner party would evaporate from her memory overnight. What's the point of fun if you can't remember it? And the sad truth is that when people catch a whiff of dementia, they back off quickly. When the party's over, they don't call back. Who can blame them?

That was particularly hard for me to watch. This was a woman who had been a social "alpha" all her life, and her charm and manners and vocabulary were hard-wired into her so thoroughly that she could still pull it together most of the time and fool people for a while. For a while. Then she'd slip, repeat something she'd just finished saying, or maybe say something peculiar about being in Connecticut, and I'd see the little moment of comprehension on peoples' faces . . .

And a deep streak of contrariness in my mother helped to nullify my efforts. Mitch was in a local play that winter. My mother often talked about joining the theatre group in town. "I'd like to try out," she said. Mitch and I zipped our lips at the notion of a woman with Alzheimer's learning lines—indeed, even remembering that she was in a play—but I took her to one of his rehearsals thinking maybe she could run lines, or make friends, or just be entertained. She sat for about fifteen minutes and then whispered that she was bored and wanted to go home.

If I took her to an informal session of singing at a local musician's house, because singing in a chorus had once been one of her great pleasures, she'd sit, silent and diffident, then whisper that she felt lousy and wanted to go home.

And writing? Forget it. My mother's prolific typewriter had always thundered away up on the top floor back home. Now it sat silent and dusty. She didn't like the action of the keys, she said (never mind that it was her own machine). So I got her another. And another. Soon she had four typewriters lined up on her desk. Plenty of paper, pencils, Wite-Out. The only thing I ever saw her write was half a letter, never finished, and the effort cost her a week of fretting and fluttering. Now *that* really scared me. Writers, beware: It's one of the first things to go.

A terrible transformation began to take place in me: embarrassment at her condition. The mother I once loved to show off because she was so much cooler and smarter than anyone else's mother. Now I scrambled to cover up the gaps, compensate, and before long, hide her.

How quickly my mother, Mitch and I became a Sartre-esque threesome. Oh, Sartre was brilliant. He could have chosen two people for his existential hell, or four, or ten, or seventy-one. But he chose three, the points of a triangle, the magic human number for maximum madness and misery.

Before we knew it, our own little No Exit clanged shut around us: My daily phone call to her, 9:00 A.M. sharp. Mitch delivering her paper, visiting with her to keep her away from me for a while so I could get some work done in the crucial morning hours. The Pittsburgh Steelers Front Four, he called himself, the line through which not even she could penetrate. Her sighs of desolation and loneliness. Her yearning to return to Connecticut and the vanished good times. Both of us trying to explain why that wasn't possible. Tears over Mike, as fresh and hot as if he had died just yesterday. My churning, muddy emotions while I desperately tried to write about plague and murder in 740 A.D. Canton, at triple speed, angst rolling around like a bowling ball in my solar plexus. I had less than six months now to do what needed a solid year, and every day I slipped a little further behind.

It became obvious right away that we'd have to hire someone or go crazy. My brother said he'd find the money. Mitch put up flyers around town: *Need help with physically vigorous but forgetful mom. Companionship, excursions, etc. Men invited to apply.* We'd actually made a couple of tentative efforts to have someone keep her company. Both times we'd got women, and my mother instantly rejected them. We knew that our chances of having her accept someone aside from one of us would be better if that person were male and reasonably presentable. An arm to hold, an escort.

Only one person responded. He was a yoga teacher as well as a caregiver. He hadn't always been in this line of work. He'd had money once, had been an entrepreneur. He'd had a spiritual awakening, though, and found his true calling—caring for the elderly and the disabled at an astoundingly affordable price. We hired him right away. His name was Allen, and without him we might all be in our graves by now. She accepted him, and he had infinite patience.

He took her out in our car, or for walks around town or to the beach, from about two o'clock until six, the dinner hour, when he delivered her to our door. She was still making her own breakfast and lunch, but dinner alone was unthinkable. There had been way too many lonely dinners with too much vodka in her big old house in Connecticut. I had pledged that there would be no more lonely nights, but I had, naturally, envisioned friends and activities . . .

I had also envisioned her strolling to the market a few blocks away in our beautiful village, doing some of her shopping for herself.

Forget that, too. She had a hard time finding her way from her apartment to our house, but she sure as hell could find her way to the liquor store at the other end of town, and even talk them into taking her Connecticut check. Which meant we had to keep her wallet empty and her checkbook and credit card away from her if she was going to spend any time at all alone at her apartment so that we could have some time alone at our house. Any buying power at all neutralized her uncertainty, and she'd set out from her apartment on foot in search of hooch. And purloining her checkbook and card and keeping her wallet empty meant that we had to do a lot of fast talking and fancy footwork and all of her shopping for her. We had to control her, we had to exert discipline on her, we had to fib and dissemble, all of it perfectly contrary to how I was accustomed all of my life to relating to my mother. It affected me the way it would if someone held a gun to my head and told me I had to skin cats or be an airline stewardess. I hated it, hated it, hated it, but I had no choice. Luckily for me, Mitch has resolve in certain areas where I do not.

We were it. Except for Allen for a few hours in the afternoon a few days a week, we were her friends and activities. We were all that stood between her and the beast of aloneness. So: dinner each and every evening, on time, at our house. My efforts to keep her occupied and entertained and out of Mitch's hair just as he kept her out of mine in the mornings. Her repertoire of conversational topics—stories from the past we could have recited in unison with her or how much she missed Mike and why did he have to die when there were so many bastards in the world who deserved to die and how she wished she could just die too. My own sorrow over Mike dredged up and renewed so that I was thinking about him and crying in the middle of the night sometimes myself. Then the requests for vodka, the explanations of why she couldn't have it, the amazing conversations that I now call M.C. Escher perpetual staircase dialogues:

"Is there any hard liquor in the house?"

"No, Mom. No hard liquor. Doctor's orders."

"I don't see what difference it makes at my age. And it settles my stomach."

"It messes up your head. You don't know where you are or who you are. Besides, we've been told (lie) that hard liquor is a dangerous mix with your antidepressants."

"Oh?"

"Yes. Very bad. And you want to get your memory back, don't you?"

"Of course I do."

"So let's try an experiment. No hard liquor for a while."

"All right. I'm willing to give it a try."

"Good! Here's some wine."

"Is there any hard liquor in the house?"

And every night, dinner on little folding tables in front of the television. CNN, *Jeopardy!*, *Win Ben Stein's Money*. We were shunted like cattle in a chute into that routine quickly; she wanted it, it diverted her, we felt compelled to defer to her, and of course we couldn't just let her sit there by herself, so we joined her. And there we were, as if we'd been doing it for a thousand years, and would be doing it for another thousand.

Then came perhaps the saddest and cruelest development of them all. The one thing that brought her a bit of contentment, the thing she'd wanted so much since Mike's death, to be a member of a household and family again, quickly became a source of fingernails-on-the-blackboard irritation to both Mitch and me: my mother, bumbling around the kitchen happily, clattering dishes, opening and shutting cupboards and drawers over and over because she couldn't remember where anything was, trying to put things away or set out the silverware. Bumping into us, standing right behind us while we cooked, her cigarette smoke curling around our eyes and noses. You learn some unpleasant things about yourself. You think your love is boundless. What you find is that it's about a half-inch thick, and underneath is a mile of churlish, petty, fretful, ungenerous irascibility.

The evenings ended with me walking her home, laying out her vitamins, cleaning her cat box. Running the tub for her while she objected like a little child.

"But I took a bath this morning!"

Here's an intimate and unhappy fact of senile dementia: Its victims become unappetizing. They don't bathe unless you make them. They'll wear dirty underwear and never wash their hair. Their fingernails and feet will be grimy. Unclean children are one thing; unclean old people are quite another. You will begin to find a person you love . . . odious. And you will hate yourself for feeling it.

And the bedtime merry-go-round conversations:

"Who are the women who are taking things out of my house?"

"No one's taking anything out of your house, Mom. Everything's safe and sound."

"Someone called me and said two women were emptying my house and putting everything in storage."

"Nope. No women are taking anything out of your house. If they were, I'd know about it. You have a housesitter. Everything's fine."

"What's my housesitter's name?"

"Wally Reynolds."

"Ah, yes. Wally Reynolds. And he's taking care of things?"

"Yep. And doing a great job."

"I'll have to go back and empty the house."

"It's mostly done, Mom. Remember? We were all there together in the fall."

"But there are books and pictures and things I want to go through."

"It's done. Mostly. We'll go back when the house sells."

"But I should empty it out before it sells."

"Not necessary. Selling a house isn't like selling a car. They don't just write a check and move in the next day. There's escrow. Two to three months. Plenty of time."

"But who are the women who are taking things out of my house?"

Having a parent with dementia in your household (if you are trying to be at all kind and don't resort to simply locking the person in the basement and throwing some food down the stairs once in a while) means that everything (and I mean everything) in your life very quickly arranges itself around the dementia. Like having a two-year-old, but with some obvious and important differences.

A two-year-old is a creature of pure will. No less willful is the person with senile dementia. But the baby has limited life experience with which to exert his will. The old person has an excess of it. Other faculties may go, but the will remains powerful. If the person is your parent, and you adored and admired that parent, you'll find yourself responding to that will just as you did when the parent was a whole, intact person. You want to please, to defer, to impress.

The process of the child becoming the parent, which is of course what happens, was bitter confusion for me. She'd been my mother, so accomplished, so generous, such good manners, so kind to me, always so lucid and sensible, that my wish to defer to her and please her and impress her—and most of all, not to lose her—only very slowly and with the stubbornest reluctance gave way to the unwelcome knowledge that I was now Mommy. And a not very good one, in my opinion. A snappish, desperate and incompetent Mommy.

I've read about the struggles of the families of public figures with Alzheimer's. I know where they're coming from—but they are not in the same world with the rest of us, I promise. For an extra dimension to the anguish, they should try helplessly watching the person they love break down like Hal the Computer while bills pile up and crush them, deadlines rush toward them like the Midnight Special, and the only time they have to work is stolen minutes here and there, whenever they can, not infrequently exhausted and hung over to the point of physical and mental collapse while their "loved one" interrupts twenty times an hour and they are striving mightily not to lash out, break things, scream. They should try it without cooks, housekeepers, gated grounds, round-the-clock professional hands-on assistance. They should try it without the sympathy of the world.

When it was just us, Mitch and I would sometimes eat in the dining room, sometimes in front of the TV, sometimes at a normal hour or sometimes at 11:00 P.M. Or he'd eat when he felt like it, and I'd eat when I felt like it. No rules, no routine. During the time my mother was with us we produced 558 dinners, on schedule, every night, without fail. Probably 557 of them in front of the TV.

And every day, without fail, she'd ask, "Am I having dinner with you tonight?" Or, a slight variation, spoken in a piteous voice that caused both me and Mitch to grind our teeth: "Is there enough food for me to eat with you tonight?" Pretty lousy acting, Mitch observed.

Sarcasm rose to my tongue. Sometimes I could check it. Sometimes I couldn't. When I couldn't, I horsewhipped myself.

"No, Mom, there's not enough food. You're going to eat cold gruel tonight, alone, in the dark."

The deadline, guilt, sorrow, relentless responsibility and no life of our own was the high-octane mix we dog-paddled around in, hearing my mother's ever-narrowing set of refrains, recited daily like the stations of the cross, each one a knife in my heart: her homesickness, her loneliness, missing Mike, and the one that ultimately made us craziest of all: her stomach.

Oh, God. Her stomach.

CHAPTER FOUR

The Belly of the Beast

There is no treatment.

So said the unfriendly gastroenterologist over the phone back in Connecticut. And I'd thought: *Oh, yeah? Wait'll I get her out to California. Just wait. We'll fix this thing. And you'll be the first on the list to get your nose rubbed in it, buddy-boy.*

The sound of my mother whistling had always been the equivalent of birdsong to me—pure concentrated essence of cheer. Mike, who could recognize hundreds of different birds by their songs, identified the catch of his life in a New York office building. He told us it was one of the first things he'd noticed when they met, when they were both working as editors for a magazine—this woman who whistled while she typed, he said. He was instantly intrigued. I knew exactly what he meant. My own ear was always alert for that sound, especially now.

My mother's new California doctor was adamant from every angle: No matter what, her drinking days are over, he said—bad for her head, bad for her stomach, bad for her life. So we were keeping her dry. I had hope. We were getting through almost entire days and occasionally even whole days with no complaints, my mother completely forgetting that anything had ever been wrong, sometimes whistling little tunes. And a switch would flip in my brain in a Pavlovian sort of way: Happy Days Are Here Again.

But sometimes, along about dinnertime, after Allen had dropped her off and we'd poured her a glass of fake wine, she'd take a sip and set it down. And she'd say: "Is there any hard liquor in the house? My stomach is upset." And the switch in my head would instantly flip back into the Despair position. Give it time, her doctor said. Be patient. It could take weeks before you see consistent results.

Weeks went by. When it became abysmally clear that abstinence was having no effect whatsoever on her stomach, we renewed our assault, vigorously. Next, the doctor did a blood test and triumphantly told us he'd found antibodies to *H. pylori*. This, of course, is the bacterium discovered in the last decade or so to be responsible for the majority of gastric ulcers. The doc was excited. You can have a chronic low-grade *H. pylori* infection, he said, not enough to give you ulcers, but enough to cause a lot of discomfort. Like nausea? I asked. Yes. Like nausea, he said. And all her other symptoms, too—cramping, bloating, pain and the rest of it.

I was thrilled. What could be more tangible than bacteria? He prescribed antibiotics, powerful and expensive. I was to give them to her every day for two weeks. Never mind that they cost hundreds of dollars. I would have paid millions. This was solid treatment, I thought. This was real. This wasn't just some vague thing like abstinence. This would definitely work. We'd finally cornered it.

Two weeks later, on the same day she'd had her final pill in the course of treatment, she was on the couch with a hot water bottle on her stomach, asking if there was a hospital in the next town.

Then the doctor tried Vitamin B-12 shots. A deficiency can mess up your stomach, he said. I took her for a series of shots. The result? Is there a hospital in the next town?

Propulsid was next. This is a prescription medicine that keeps food moving out of the stomach. Sometimes the stomachs of elderly people get sluggish, he said. Food just sits there and you get nauseated. Her symptoms sound exactly like that condition. We got some. I gave it to her faithfully. I waited. A solid month of Propulsid might as well have been a month of cotton candy.

She was even tested for Lyme disease. Negative. She'd already had an endoscopy, X-rays, a CAT scan back in Connecticut. The doctor couldn't think of any other tests to give her, and he was starting to wear thin. Eventually he stopped returning our phone calls. He did do one last thing: He wrote her a prescription for medical marijuana, quasi-legal in our county since the passage of Proposition 215. People taking chemotherapy who can't keep their food down sometimes find marijuana to be a wonderful palliative. Of course, we had plenty of less-than-legal sources; pot is to northern California as corn is to Kansas. But the official stuff is strong and comparatively cheap. Since its legality is still experimental, this is not a prescription you fill at the local pharmacy; you must go to the Cannabis Club in the county seat. Mitch took her on the three-hour round-trip. He said it was like going to a speakeasy.

My mother willingly smoked the joints we rolled (not, by the way, for the first time in her life). We'd watch. "I don't feel a thing," she'd say, and a few minutes later she'd be whistling a tune. Alas, though it improved her mood for a while, it didn't really help her stomach—but it certainly helped ours.

So it was back to the alternative side of the tracks. I doggedly kept on giving her digestive enzymes and stomach-soothing teas. I kept her off dairy products. I read everything I could find in books on alternative treatments. She had Chinese herbal medicines, she had bitter evil-smelling witch's brew leaves-and-bark concoctions we made in the pressure cooker. I took her to two acupuncturists. Anyone who's had acupuncture knows that lying still and being patient are essential to the procedure. They stick the pins in you and then go away for twenty or thirty minutes. For most of us, this enforced quiet and stillness is bliss. You lie there and drift. For my mother, who'd been impatient all her life anyway and now couldn't remember the reason why she was lying on that table in the first place, it was impossible. She'd sit up, bristling with needles, and yell my name.

For naught, for naught. Sometimes we had a few days' respite from stomach complaints and thought we'd found the cure, but always, always, it came roaring back. Sometimes there were acute attacks when she'd cry and tremble and double over with pain. It was torture for me to watch her suffer and be unable to do a thing about it.

She'd beg for a drink. I was impaled. It didn't take long for us to see that keeping her dry was not going to restore her memory, either, but that didn't mean we could just say okay, never mind, bottoms up. If giving her a drink made her happy, or soothed her, I would have done it, believe me—but it didn't. Even a small one magnified her brain damage, put her in a never-never land of disorientation and fear. Alzheimer's and booze are a bad combination, let me tell you. That night at the Safeway was a vivid demonstration that letting her drink would be nothing less than cruel and negligent. I admit that I caved in a couple of times out of desperation and also to experiment. Maybe it helped her stomach once upon a time, but it didn't anymore.

Mitch and I argued. He believed that some of the time her pain was real, but that there might be other times when she faked it—not necessarily consciously, but reflexively, he theorized—to get my attention and sympathy, to get a drink. Some old acting instinct kicking in. I said, Maybe, it sure seems that way sometimes, you might be right—but what if it IS real? I can't afford NOT to believe it's real. Imagine yourself senile, I said, and suffering, and everyone around you sick of hearing about it and ignoring you. It's a thought not to be borne.

And of course, I was getting sick of hearing about it. Her complaints, her face gray with pain, her confusion, her questions about doctors, hospitals and pharmacists, verbatim virtually every day as if we'd never discussed the topic before, became the components of purgatory for us all. She'd groan, stagger, weep, hold her stomach. As the months progressed, and nothing we tried worked, I came to live in a chronic state of rage and helplessness—rage at my failure, helplessness in the face of this infuriating, baffling stomach monster that wrecked any chance at all of making my mother's life even a little bit pleasanter. It was bad enough that she had to lose her mind; it was intolerable that she should also suffer physically almost all the time, that nothing could be done, that she couldn't understand or remember how hard we'd tried, that even her doctor didn't want to hear about it anymore, that Mitch and I got so raw with impatience that we could barely stand to hear another word about it. It was a nattering nightmare. Don't take it out on her, don't take it out on her, I rebuked myself. Don't. Don't.

But sometimes I did. Not that I beat her or anything crude like that. I promise I didn't. But there were times when I snapped at her, yelled, stamped my foot or clenched my fists and hissed with poisonous exasperation. Mitch, my valiant trooper most of the time, raised his voice (and he has quite a voice) more than once. She'd cry: I wish I could just die. If I had a gun I'd shoot myself.

Then would come remorse and more self-flagellation. Was this what my mother deserved, in her sickness and loss? To be at the mercy of a couple of unsympathetic ill-tempered louts like us? Had I really, really tried everything to help her, or was I just giving up because I'm too selfish and stupid and lazy to find the cure? She, who had always come to my rescue in my misspent youth, and ever so recently, in my misspent middle age? I felt hard and mean and full of sorrow all at once, and it drove me truly mad. Drove me, in fact, to drink.

At the beginning, when we first told her she'd have to stay off the vodka, we were honorable and upright. If we were going to ask her to abstain, then so would we. Such integrity! In just a couple of months, we were the ones with hidden bottles. We moved like sorcerers, deftly bringing out the hooch while she was right there in the room with us and her attention was diverted for a moment, pouring ourselves stiff ones and drinking them nonchalantly out of coffee cups right in front of her. Sometimes in the middle of the day. Sometimes in the morning, something I'd never done before in my life.

I discovered a wee shot at dawn to be the best way to shut down my poor roiling head and get back to sleep for another hour or two. I found zen-like little oases of peace and solitude, propped on my pillow and staring into my soft red night-light at 6 A.M., sipping from a cup, feeling the alcohol spreading its soothing tentacles from my stomach to my limbs and brain, displacing the residue from an unpleasant dream. Like this one: I'm at my mother's house in Connecticut. Mike has come back to life for a while, just a while, we all know it's only temporary, and he and my mother are stripping the house bare, even taking down the walls.

I met Mike for the first time in the front hall of my mother's house. It was summer, 1966. I was home from boarding school. My mother had gone to New York about a year before to work at *American Heritage* magazine. That's where she and Mike found each other, where he noticed the amazing Whistling Typing Woman. She came up to Connecticut on weekends and whenever else she could. I was on my own at the house that summer, and this time she brought the new man in her life with her.

He was young and had a sandy beard and hair and blue eyes. And even though I was a sullen, smirky self-centered teenager steeped in adolescent ennui, I liked him instantly. He put out his right hand in an eager, friendly way. The hand was red and smallish. I'd see him do that a million times over the next twenty-three years—offer the hand immediately to a new person, as if to say: Here it is, let's get it over with.

He was born with vascular anomalies in his right arm. It was a little shorter than the entirely normal left arm, and there was a birthmark over most of it called a hemangioma, commonly known as a "port wine" mark. He'd had circulation problems with the arm all his life. There had been talk of amputating it when he was a child, but they didn't, and since he was right-handed he worked the arm to strengthen it. And he worked at overcoming his self-consciousness as well. That's why he always offered the hand first thing. Most people didn't notice the hand, but Mike once said it was on his mind every moment of every day.

With the exception of my father, my mother's choice of men in her active and complicated love life had been marked by an unfortunate susceptibility to style rather than content. She knew it, lamented it, wrote about it in her fiction. With the advent of Mike, my mother entered an era where style took on an entirely new and mature definition. This time, style and content were inseparable. Mike was handsome, but not in the flashy, obvious way Durant (and others too numerous to mention) had been. His beard compensated for a chin that was weak compared to the rest of his head, which was large, with an open and wonderfully pleasant face. His physique was entirely ordinary, and he had to pay attention to a waist that always wanted to expand. And there was the arm.

Mike was a direct descendant of the great abolitionist William Lloyd Garrison. If a powerful social conscience is genetic, then Mike carried a wheelbarrow of his ancestor's genes. And just as Durant had encouraged certain unfortunate character flaws in my mother, with Mike, her best qualities—humor, generosity, responsibility, flexibility, reasonableness, breadth of vision, lucidity—flourished. She felt loved, really loved, at last. And the fact that she was twelve years older than he mattered not a whit to him. He never, ever, not once in all their years together said or did anything to make her feel old or to make her feel that she was anything less than beautiful and desirable. What a man. I shall not look upon his like again.

And funny? Christ, we used to laugh our fool heads off. There's no tonic more exhilarating for body and soul than helpless laughter. He loved to have a good story told on him. One of the best was one they brought back from the Audubon trip. They'd been camping some-where—Labrador, I think—and my mother was mixing them a couple of drinks by the fire in the early evening. My mother saw a forest ranger approaching to say howdy. They were on a beach, so there were no snapping twigs or crunching leaves to announce the man's arrival. Mike had his back to the guy, and didn't see him, because he was looking at my mother and the drinks clinking in her hands. And he said, in his fun. playful way: "Dinky for Mikey?" This was a private joke, a reference to a pet word for evening cocktails used by some elderly relative of his, and which my mother and Mike sometimes invoked to entertain each other. The ranger, of course, didn't know this, but heard it loud and clear. Too late, Mike saw the expression on my mother's face, turned and saw the ranger, and the incident entered the annals of history. For years after that, when my mother handed him a drink, she'd occasionally say, "Dinky for Mikey?" and we'd all be instantly weak with hilarity, especially Mike.

When he was a boy, he'd wanted to change his name, he told us—to Lance. He'd liked the rugged masculine sound of it: Lance Harwood. We were convulsed, and Mike shook his head incredulously. Not too Freudian or anything, he said. Not too phallic. That, too, entered the archives. When I sent him something in the mail after that I'd sometimes address it in big letters to Lance Harwood. Or when I called on the phone and he answered, I'd say: Mr. Lance Harwood, please. And we'd roar. I loved Mike so much. He used to sign his letters to me Y.M.O.S.D.: Your Mean Old Step Dad.

My mother told me once that if she ever got run over by a bus, I was to destroy a certain secret box of letters and journals so that Mike wouldn't have to see them. She showed me where she'd cleverly hidden them. Why did she keep them? Not for sentimental reasons, that's for sure. She kept them because she was a writer, and writers have a tendency to keep potentially risky stuff around. It wasn't that Mike would be angry, or jealous, or would make a scene if he saw it. She just didn't want to hurt him with graphic glimpses of her heavily populated past sex life. Mike had been married before, but he was an innocent compared to my mother.

They escaped New York together permanently around 1970, moving to Connecticut to get married and live happily ever after. And for a good long time, they did. The town quickly fell in love with Mike. When he died, my mother got at least a thousand letters from grieving friends and even people who'd only met him once or twice. It was a tide, a torrent, and it lifted and carried her. Why is grief easier to bear when it's shared? It's a mystery. But it's so.

Connecticut. Her wit, her intellect, her creativity all erode away like desert sandstone while Connecticut stands solid in her memory.

"I think I'll go back to Connecticut and live with Joan Talbridge."

"Mom, you can't go live with Joan Talbridge."

"Why not?"

"Because she has a life of her own. She can't take care of you. She's not your family."

"I don't think I need to be taken care of."

"But you do. Your memory's full of holes. You need to be with your family."

"Joan invited me to come live with her."

"She invited you for a visit. Not to live with her. To visit. She can't do the job that a family does."

"Give me some examples of some of these goofy things I'm supposed to have done."

"Well, the fact that we've already had this conversation about fifty times is one example."

"No, really. Give me some examples."

Deep breath.

"Well, you were bilked out of almost eight grand. You couldn't find your way to old friends' houses where you'd been going for forty years. You had to carry a map of the town around in your car. You were depressed and crying whenever I called you on the phone. You called me once to say you'd taken Polly to a kennel, but you couldn't remember which one, so you called all of them and none of them had her, and then it turned out Polly was shut in the basement. Every one of your old friends was worried about you. They called me and Tommy up to tell us they were worried about you."

"They were worried about me?"

"Yes. All of them. Because of little things that were adding up. Joan Talbridge was one of the people who was worried about you."

"Give me some examples."

Breathe again.

"I just did. That's an example."

"I could go live with Joan Talbridge."

My mother had a little blue car, a Toyota sedan. We left it in Connecticut with André, our oldest, closest friend, when she came to California. We weren't sure what its fate would be. Maybe André would like to use it, maybe we'd sell it. Taking the car keys away from someone with Alzheimer's can be a big, big problem. We got off easy on that one. Instead of taking the car away from my mother, we took my mother away from the car.

A couple of months after she'd arrived, André called and said a young acquaintance, an Israeli fellow traveling around the U.S., would like to drive her car to California. Okay, we said. We still weren't sure what we'd do with it. Maybe Allen would drive her around in it. Maybe we'd sell it. But we'd have it. And here was a way to transport two more of her typewriters, big heavy upright office machines that we'd left in her house. Even if she never used them, if they just ended up sitting on her desk looking familiar, I wanted them. They were HER typewriters, magnificent old sturdy reliable things. She'd put a lot of miles on both of them. So the Israeli put the two typewriters in my mother's car and set out on his cross-country journey.

Somewhere deep in the heart of Texas, the car threw a rod because somebody along the way failed to replace the oil cap. The Israeli called André, who called us. The car was towed to a garage. The Israeli got on a plane and continued on his way.

The mechanic in Texas said the car was not worth fixing, but that he'd pay us a couple of hundred and use it for parts. He'd need the title, though, before he could pay us.

The title was somewhere in my mother's house. Buried in her study, no doubt. André made a foray there, but it was hopeless. One piece of paper in a room jammed with fifty thousand pieces of paper? Forget it.

My brother said he'd write to the Connecticut DMV and get a replacement. The Texas guy said that was fine, he was in no hurry. Meantime, what about these here typewriters? How 'bout if I ship 'em to you and take the cost off what I pay you for the car? It's a deal, we said.

About a week later, the UPS truck dropped off two big boxes. I opened one. There was my mother's old Royal, sitting there with no packing of any kind. No newspaper, no Styrofoam peanuts, no nothing. The carriage return and ribbon mechanism were smashed and dented as if the typewriter had been in a head-on collision. The Texas mechanic had simply put the typewriter in the box, taped it shut, and sent it. It was the same with the other one.

I raged. You moron. You stupid, stupid fucking jackass moron. You call yourself a mechanic? I thought of her car, her little blue car with the Connecticut plates, her little car that had once whizzed along green Connecticut roads, in a junkyard in Texas, and now her typewriters, carelessly tossed in boxes like more junk, dented, bent, smashed, ruined. More of her life dismantled, lost, plowed under. I raged, and I knelt on the floor over the typewriters and sobbed.

I took them to our best fix-it guy, but he said they were a lost cause. I couldn't bear to just throw them away. My mother's typewriters! And I didn't want her to see them all smashed up. I thought of vaguely ceremonial ways to dispose of them. Burial at sea? A sort of Viking funeral, perhaps? Then I had a brilliant, truly inspired idea. One night after dark I put the typewriters in my car and left them outside the back door of the local theatre. They could pass as props. Even bent and broken, they could still pretend to be typewriters.

January: She's been with us just a little over two months. I hide in the dark about forty feet from the double sliding glass kitchen door of our house. It's cold, so I'm dressed warmly—big overcoat, sweater, socks. I wait. My heart pounds with fury, sorrow, anguish. I sit cross-legged, leaning against a wooden outbuilding in our ninety-year-old neighbor's yard. I'm nestled way back in the ivy, deep in the shadows. The light from our kitchen casts itself partway across the yard, but I imagine looking out from the inside and know he won't be able to see me.

He? Mitch. A while before, he had done that thing that men allow themselves to do—stomped out of the house in a rage and slammed the door. We had a big fight over how I hadn't got my mother out of there and back to her apartment a block away with enough dispatch after dinner that evening. Anyway, WHAM went the door and he was gone into the night.

I'll be fucked, I thought, if I'll just sit here like a woman and wait for him to come back. When he does, I won't be here. He can wonder where I am. So, in a big hurry, I'd bundled up and hustled out the door. But I wasn't going to go walk the streets the way he was surely doing. Uh-uh. I was going to put myself where I could spy on him when he got back to the house. I was going to see what he did when he came in and discovered I wasn't there. I'd find a place where I could watch, and I would wait.

I wait. And wait. The cold starts to penetrate my warm clothes, and my legs are getting stiff, and I rearrange myself a lot, but I wait.

I'm shaking, teeth clattering, but still out there when I hear the front door again almost an hour later.

The living room's not visible from my hiding place, but the kitchen with its double glass doors is practically like a stage set. He comes in, opens the refrigerator for a beer, obviously assuming that I'm up in bed or something. Goes back into the living room. Stays in there for a while, twenty minutes at least. Go look for me, you rotten son of a bitch, I mutter. I want to see you look for me.

Eventually he goes upstairs. I see the bedroom light flick on and then off quickly. First surprise. Ha!

He comes down, carrying Otto, our big old orange cat. Opens the kitchen door, puts Otto out. Then he gets a flashlight, comes out the glass doors, goes to the studio in the backyard. After a minute he comes back to the house. Surprise number two. I'm shaking harder, now not just from cold but from elation. He's actually searching for me. He grabs keys from the hook in the kitchen. He's out the front door again. I hear it shut. I know what he's doing: He's walking over to my mother's apartment to see if I'm there. I picture him stealthily unlocking the door, creeping up the carpeted stairs with a flashlight, the beam searching the living room. Surprise number three.

He's back in five minutes. I see him lean his forehead tiredly against the refrigerator for a moment. The actions of a man who does not know he is being watched. I decide I'll make him wait a little longer.

Not too long, though, soft-hearted wretch that I am.

CHAPTER FIVE

Heart of Glass

She'd been with us six months, and we were moving. We decided that it would be easier on us and on her to have her on the same property but in her own little house. Far from the liquor store. We were running back and forth between her apartment and our rented house ten times a day, and when I was at home I could feel the force field of her loneliness, like something alive, emanating from the direction of her apartment—loneliness and its close compatriot, uselessness.

We bought a house, my brother arranging the incredibly complex financing from afar, betting heavily on the eventual sale of the house in Connecticut. I was still struggling with the novel, three more chapters to go, so Mitch had to handle most of the move. He was game and dauntless, but until you start tearing apart, under extreme duress, a place where two packrats have denned for five full years you can't really know what you're in for.

And we were tearing up the little apartment, too, after a scant six months. She was supposed to love it, but she didn't. She didn't love it at all. Talk about a gilded cage. The beauty of the place—the ocean view, the flower garden, her books and pictures, the town itself—had taken on a tragic, deceitful quality. It wasn't Connecticut. It wasn't home. And she wasn't even sure what home she was missing. Sometimes she'd say: *I can't picture the house I lived in.* Suppressing a little subterranean ripple of terror,

I'd describe it: the road, the front door, the view from the back porch.
She'd listen, eyes squeezed shut. Sometimes it would pop back into her
head, and sometimes it wouldn't. And sometimes she'd ask me about
another house, her family's summer home from her childhood, on the
lake in the same Connecticut town. No, Mom, I'd say, you sold that house
fifty years ago.

It was too sad. She couldn't always remember the place she was missing, but that didn't stop her from being in an acute state of longing,
which only intensified as she struggled to recall the image of home.
Slipping away, slipping away. The farther it slipped, the more she
yearned. And I was the one who'd taken her away. I had deprived her of
the place and the memory of it.

Now the apartment would slip into history, too. The lease was up,
so we moved her out, scrubbed and cleaned, and stashed her temporarily in the run-down little studio in the backyard of the old house. There
was no explaining any of this to her. Not that it mattered much—she
forgot the apartment instantly. It had never existed.

I sat in my ransacked study and wrote for a few hours every day
while Mitch tramped past my door a hundred times carrying furniture
and huge boxes and my mother wandered in and out, confusion multiplying logarithmically in her head as the chaos grew around us.
Somehow, mostly thanks to Mitch, the manuscript got finished. The circumstances under which I had to work affected the result, I believe in
a positive way. It's a tale of desperation that needed to race along. It's
desperate, and it races along. I got paid, but of course that money lasted
about five minutes because we owed so much already. We paid a few
bills, but then the drought resumed with renewed ferocity.

We worked for days with no sleep, stuffing boxes into the car like
fleeing refugees, making trip after trip after trip, my mother riding with
us, asking anxious questions over and over. We moved her into the master bedroom of the new house while Mitch and I, a couple of stumbling
zombies, burrowed in among piles of books and clothing in the spare
room. Meanwhile, a carpenter was converting the garage into a "granny
unit" for my mother, Mitch helping, pushing things along, ordering and
hauling supplies, my brother again handling the financing from afar. As

soon as that unit is finished, we told ourselves, everything will be fine. No more running back and forth between house and apartment in town. She'll be snug in her own little place and we'll be just a few steps away.

One evening shortly after we moved in, Mitch made a little joke to my mother about "room service" when he brought her a snack on a tray. She laughed, accepted the snack and pretended to tip him. Ah ha, I thought. A little moment of normalcy, for which I was pathetically grateful. She'd been famous for her sense of humor. She and my brother and I used to get into giggling fits in forbidden places—weddings and concerts and such.

The next morning, my mother was dressed and sitting on the window seat in the living room.

"There's no need to stay here any longer," she said. "We should check out now."

I was barefoot, in my bathrobe, hair mashed, a Breathe Right stuck to my nose.

"Where," I asked cautiously, "do you think we are?"

I saw a flash of fear in her eyes.

"Isn't this a hotel?"

The independence we envisioned for her at the new place, which would also be the solution to her awful, devouring loneliness—her own little house ten feet away from ours—turned out to be our worst delusion so far. She'll know we're right there, we thought, and enjoy her cozy little home on this lovely piece of land, with its own TV and kitchen and bathroom . . .

She became our prisoner, and we became hers, in a way that made the endless winter before the move seem like a tiptoe through the tulips.

She lived under the same roof with us for about six weeks before the cottage was habitable. The house has a great big kitchen and dozens of cupboards. She had done a lot of cupboard-banging back in the kitchen at the old house, searching for utensils whose location she could never learn, and it had annoyed us a lot, but now she was like a musician going from a small electronic keyboard to a mighty church organ. There are thirty-six cupboard doors in the kitchen, each with a slightly different pitch. Mitch and I lay in bed in our junk-packed little room at dawn or the middle of the night listening to the symphony: BANGETY-BANG BANG BANG! BANG! BANGETY-BANG!

This banging was a sound wired into my system from the more distant past as well, all the way back to childhood in Connecticut. My mother when she was young and whole had an impressive temper, and cupboard noise was one of its expressions. Now, decades later, every BANG sent shock waves of mingled associations, one ancient and primal and the other recently acquired, along my worn and frazzled nerves and up to my brain—DONG!—like one of those strong-man apparatuses at the carnival. It was around then that I noticed myself getting seriously jumpy. I flinched and twitched and leapt at any small unanticipated noise, or if Mitch came around a corner when I wasn't expecting him, or worst of all, when my mother called my name.

The money my brother had set aside for the garage conversion ran out, naturally, before the work was quite finished. The walls were up and the plumbing and electricity were in, but Mitch and I did all the taping and mudding and then the sanding ourselves. (Loads of fun—fine white powder in every orifice and follicle of your head, raining down into your eyes, mouth and nose while you sand the ceiling with a device on the end of a long pole, arms aching, working till well after midnight night after night, drinking, radio blaring.) After that we primed and painted the walls, then scrubbed and scraped the cement floor, primed and painted it. Then we lugged furniture, rugs, books, put up curtains, all at top speed. My mother would wander in and out, admire the work, compliment us. "This is going to be your little house, Mom," I'd tell her, brightly, guiltily, but it rolled right off her. I don't think it was merely a matter of faulty memory—I think she just plain didn't want to hear it. She'd wander away, then come back five minutes later.

"Tell me again," she'd say. "Why are you doing all this?"

The night finally came when we moved her into the cottage. I felt as if I were putting her out on an ice floe. Stability and predictability, chant the experts. This, including the move from her house in Connecticut, was move number four in seven months.

Mitch disconnected her porch light and switched ours off so all she saw from the lighted interior was India ink. This time, he and I crouched in the dark together, hiding behind the car, watching my mother move around inside her new house, pacing, peering out the windows, her eyes alert but blank and dead all at once, a look we'd come to know too well. We were exultant. She's in! We did it! Our new era begins! I had laid out everything she'd need for breakfast, shown it all to her: oatmeal, honey, tea, butter, bread, eggs, bananas, all utensils. Milk, bacon and orange juice in the refrigerator. She had a hot plate, a sink, a toaster, a blender. Polly nested happily on the sofa. Familiar pictures on the wall, fresh sheets on the bed—she could be near us, part of the family, but independent! The last six weeks had been intolerably intimate, with no apartment to send her to, *nowhere* to send her to, but now, at last, she was in her new home, autonomous but not alone.

Early the next morning, I woke to cupboards banging. I flew out of bed and down the hall to the kitchen. She was in her nightgown, barefoot, bewildered. She was looking for something to eat.

August: We're riding in the Volvo, which needs new tires, a new steering rack and a new muffler. She's always in the car with me, because she wants to go with me everywhere I go. It's impossible to get to the car and out the driveway without her seeing me. Sometimes I'm able to sneak away by going out the side door of the house, hunching over and crawling in the passenger side of the car, but I usually get busted. There's nothing at all wrong with her eyes and ears. I'm alone all the time, she says. Alone and staring at the wall. Reminding her that she's in fact rarely alone, except for a few hours in the morning (if I'm lucky), does no good. In her mind, she's alone all the time.

My clothes are not particularly clean. Neither are my mother's. Her hair needs washing. Mine does too, but not as obviously as hers. She gives off an aroma, not exactly offensive, but slightly . . . zoological. And complex: It contains elements of her old scent from long ago that had intoxicated me when I was a child. Cologne, cigarette smoke, lipstick. I used to smell the clothes in her closet and swoon a little. Now it's those old nostalgic smells mixed with this peculiar geriatric animal smell. In the close atmosphere of the car, the mix of olfactory messages confuses my poor brain.

"What was the name of the doctor I saw last time I was out here?" my mother asks. Her tone is normal, conversational. A person riding with us for the first time would find nothing out of the ordinary in her question. But if that person were also watching my hands on the steering wheel, he or she might have noticed them whitening. If I were hooked up to a blood-pressure monitor and an EKG, the technicians would sit up in alarm.

I keep my own voice as calm and normal as I can.

"It wasn't last time, Mom. You've been out here for almost a year. You've been to five doctors since you've been here."

"And none of them had any suggestions?"

"You've got them all stumped, Mom."

"You'd think in this day and age they could solve a simple stomach problem."

"Well," I say, the gravitational pull sucking me in, "less than a century ago they didn't even have antibiotics, or anesthesia. They held you down or hit you over the head while they sawed your leg off. Medicine is actually still kind of primitive." A few years back, such a comment would have provoked a lively discussion with my intellectually nimble mother. Instead:

"Have I been to a gastroenterologist?"

"You've been to the best from coast to coast."

"And none of them had anything to say."

"They've given you every test there is, Mom. You've had CAT scans, MRIs, endoscopies, blood tests. They can't find anything wrong."

"There was a pharmacist in the next town. He gave me something that worked." She points vaguely to the northeast through the car window.

"No, Mom. There's no next town. Nothing's worked. If there were something that worked I'd have a truckload of it. I'd be giving it to you night and day."

"This happened the last time I was out here."

"No. No. There was no 'last time.' You've been here for a year. Your stomach's been bothering you for three years now. No one can figure it out. It's got nothing to do with being out here."

"It didn't happen back home."

Now the blood-pressure and EKG technicians would be on their feet.

"No, Mom, no! It started years ago. At home. You went to three different gastroenterologists in Connecticut. You went to the hospitals all over the state. You went to five hundred doctors. No one can find anything physically wrong."

"What was the name of the doctor I saw last time I was out here?"

When she had her apartment in town, she was constrained somewhat by not being completely sure how to get to our house. No more! The front door to the new house bursts open twenty, thirty, forty times a day, every day: my mother, searching for her basket (which she carries instead of a purse, always has), asking if she's having dinner with us, showing us a grocery list, asking if there's vodka in the house, telling us she's going to take a nap, asking the name of the doctor she saw last time she was here, showing us a grocery list, searching for her basket, telling us she wishes she knew when she was going to die, asking if there's vodka in the house, showing us a grocery list, asking if there's a hospital in the next town, telling us she's going to take a nap, asking the name of the doctor she saw last time she was here, asking if she's having dinner with us, telling us she wishes she knew when she was going to die, asking if there's a hospital in the next town, asking if there's vodka in the house, searching for her basket.

Searching for her basket. We hear many things repeated countless thousands of times, but the hands-down winner, the one that will surely earn her a spot in the *Guinness Book of World Records'* Most Frequently Asked Question category would have to be: "Where's my basket?" It becomes code for Mitch and me as we come to believe that we ourselves are hopping down the bunny trail of dementia. In some small moment of chaos or insanity I look at him, or he looks at me, and one of us mutters: "Where's my basket?"

Oh, yes. You do get involved. You become an inmate in your own private asylum for the Genteel Insane. You find yourself doing things like putting a sign out in the driveway, at your mother's behest, with big black bold-face letters reading: "DINNER PARTY TONIGHT CAN-CELED!" when no dinner party was even planned.

Why? Because she'd come into the house after waking up from a nap insisting that she'd invited a big group of people to dinner, but that we had no food, and so we had to do something to head them off.

Arguing is useless.

"No one's coming for dinner, Mom. If they were, I'd know about it."

Uh-uh. Forget it. Much easier, much more expedient, as I finally get through my thick head, is to find a big piece of cardboard and a Magic Marker, let her help set up the sign with bricks and a folding chair. Then she can relax, and then she'll forget. Then I can slip out later and remove the sign. End of story until the next time.

Sometimes, amazingly enough, we actually do round up sympathetic people and have dinner parties. She rises to the occasion, has a good time, talking, sometimes dancing, doing what she loves best—socializing. I see her in a tête-à-tête with someone, and my heart gives a little surge of joy. When the guests are gone, she sighs.

"Well, that was certainly a strange evening. No one said hello to me. No one acknowledged me or spoke one word to me. I just sat there by myself for the entire party."

My heart plummets, my voice rises. In an instant, I am the child wanting to make my mother happy, and I've failed.

"What do you mean? How can you say that? People were all over you. You were the life of the party. That's crazy."

She shrugs, makes a skeptical little noise out of the side of her mouth just as she's done as long as I've known her, and gazes away from me, forlorn and pathetic.

Breathe, I tell myself. Breathe.

She still whistles occasionally. And sings. One of her favorites is a refrain from a Sinatra song: *She hates California, it's cold and it's damp!* She thinks it's funny, snaps her fingers while she sings it, just about every day now. We listen with faces of stone.

Breathe, Mitch and I tell ourselves. Breathe.

* * *

September: I'm sitting at the computer in my "study," a room in a far corner of the house jammed with clothes, papers, books, unpaid bills. A tap-tap on the door nearly sends me out of my skin. The floorboards do not creak. They give no warning at all.

"El-Belle?" Her pet name for me. One of the sweetest sounds in the world once. Now I leap as if someone had fired a gun in the hall.

I summon a pleasant tone. "I'm right here," I say.

"Listen, dear. I have a problem." She comes in and shuts the door, leans back against it, smoking a cigarette. She looks and sounds so absolutely normal. "Some woman came and borrowed all my letters from home and hasn't brought them back."

I close my eyes and gather myself together before I answer.

"No one took your letters, Mom. They're all out there in your cottage."

"No. There was a woman who came and took them."

"Now, why would someone do a thing like that?"

"She visited me, and I showed her the letters, and she said she'd like to take them and read them."

"Mom, if someone had come here, I'd know about it. I seriously doubt there was any woman who took your letters."

"No, there was a woman."

"What was her name? What did she look like?" Here I go. That old gravitational pull. Arguing with a memory-damaged person is, without a doubt, one of the meanest, stupidest things you can do. Like challenging a paraplegic to a footrace.

"Her name starts with a 'C.' It's an odd name. That's why I can't remember it. 'C-r-e-e' something or other."

"You can't remember it because she doesn't exist." I despise the churlish, overbearing tone of my voice. My mother defends herself bravely.

"She came here when you were gone. She wanted to interview me for the newspaper. She wanted to know about where I came from, so I gave her the letters."

"Mom, if someone were going to interview you I'd sure as hell know about it."

"Well, she took them."

"No, she didn't."

"Yes, she did."

"She doesn't exist." I feel cruel. It's a powerful compulsion. I try to get a grip. "They're here. You've misplaced them. I'll help you look for them later. I think there's just been a misunderstanding."

"Well," she says, my conciliatory words apparently helping her save some face, "we'll see if you can find them. I can't."

"I'll find them."

"They were in a big manila envelope."

"I'm sure I can find them."

This is maybe the fifteenth time we've had this conversation, a couple of times already that day, and it's my fault, because I haven't done what I know I should, what Mitch has told me I must do: Gather up a bunch of her unanswered letters from home (there are dozens and dozens of them), put them in a big manila envelope, and tell her they've been returned. Breathe life into the imaginary woman, too, if I must. Describe her hair and clothing. You learn that this is what you have to do. Truth is sometimes worse than useless.

On that first morning when she came into the house looking for food, I gently steered her back out to the cottage and showed her all her breakfast stuff. "You should have your breakfast out here, Mom," I'd say. "It's easier. Then dinner with us tonight, just like every night!" It worked for a while, maybe a month or two. Sometimes she didn't emerge until eleven or so. A few precious hours for me to try to work, to give Mitch a break—though of course I felt guilty every millisecond: over her, over Mitch. The universe had served up the perfect, custom-tailored dilemma for me—to try to make two people happy, each at the expense of the other. I'm so faintheartedly bad at this sort of balancing act that it's the reason I never signed up for call-waiting. Imagine, then, how it was for me to be caught, day after deteriorating day, between the escalating needs of two people I desperately love—my man and my poor damaged mother.

But by then, guilt was my familiar old pal, a big heavy hairy arm draped around my shoulders twenty-four hours a day, and I was learning to live with it. We encouraged her to make her lunch out there, too. It was a simple lunch, the same one she'd made every day by rote for years. I always stocked her little kitchen with the necessary ingredients. That worked for a while, too. Then she started carrying her lunch stuff into the house, clattering around the kitchen.

"I was hoping I could have lunch with you," she'd say, using the same piteous voice she used when she asked if there was enough food for her to have dinner with us. "I'm alone all the time."

This was my mother. What was I to do? Was I to say, "No, Mom. Take your food and march back out to your cottage and cook there and leave us alone!!" Mitch occasionally succeeded in turning her around, firmly and usually kindly, but it was almost impossible for me.

Soon I was cooking lunch for her, because she was forgetting even this routine, making weird disturbing blunders like trying to boil water in the cat dish or make oatmeal in the ashtray, putting the ingredients for spinach soup in her electric teapot instead of her blender and scorching the whole mess. Then she began to creep in at breakfast. Often she couldn't remember if she'd eaten it or not, though I still faithfully laid out her food and utensils every night. I'd have to go out and look.

Sometimes she hadn't, so I'd make it for her. And thus it went, until I was cooking for her three times a day. I'd pretty much petered out on the brain nutrients and vitamins by then. They were expensive, made no difference at all, and represented one more disheartening routine. I did hang in there with the antidepressants, but I might as well have thrown crumpled balls of tissue paper into a raging furnace.

She spent less and less time in her cottage. She lay on the window seat in our house, sometimes complaining about her stomach and asking about doctors all the livelong day. She didn't cry often when I was a child, but when she did, it devastated me. Now she'd cry three or four times an hour, suddenly and with no warning, and my old reflexes kicked in each time. God, the perversity of her disease. Everything that made her a whole person was going, going, gone, but the memory of Mike and his death grew steadily sharper and newer every day.

"Why did Mike have to die?" she'd sob. "When I think of all the bastards who deserve to die." I'd feel my own eyes bulging with tears. *Mike, Mike.* Then it would pass as abruptly as it began, a little tropical squall, and in the next moment she'd be whistling a tune. I, helpless, was jerked this way and that by every rise, fall, zig and zag of her emotions.

We'd give her a Lorazepam, a sedative prescribed by her doctor, and try to get her to go out and take a nap in the cottage. She'd go, usually acting like a beaten puppy being put out in the rain. We'd watch her pull her curtains, and we'd look at each other and wait. Sometimes we'd get a whole hour. Usually we'd get about five minutes, ten on a good day. We didn't call her Rasputina for nothing. Her vigor was frightening. A dose that would have knocked me flat barely fazed her. We'd hear steps, then the front door would burst open. The door of her house in Connecticut was big and heavy and tended to stick. You had to throw your weight against it when you went in. The door at the new house didn't stick at all, but her habit of forty years did. She came through it like a narcotics agent every time: WHAM!

One morning I'm awake before dawn, up for a few minutes to let the cats out before I go back to bed, everything peaceful and silent. The door bursts open. I jump at least two feet off the floor and my heart nearly stops.

My mother, fully dressed, carrying her basket. She had awakened in the dark, looked at the clock, thought it was six in the evening and time for dinner.

"If I need to be taken care of, why didn't you come back and live in Connecticut? Why did I have to come out here?"

It's a blazing sunny day. We're sitting out on the deck.

"Mom, if I went back and lived in Connecticut I'd go crazy."

"Why?"

"I'm not twenty-five anymore, Mom. You think of me as twenty-five, but I'm not. If I went back there I'd feel old. I feel young out here."

"You couldn't feel young in Connecticut?"

"No. God, no. I'd feel time speeding up. I'd be old before my foot touched the ground."

"How old are you now?"

"Take a guess."

"Oh—thirty-five?"

"I wish," I snort.

"Why would you feel old in Connecticut?"

"Oh, God. Where do I begin? For one thing, the seasons are too distinct. They rush by like a speeded-up slideshow. Summer, fall, winter, spring. Summer, fall, winter, spring. It's relentless. You can never forget how fast time is going by. It's a little easier to forget about that out here."

"But you had a good time growing up there."

"Yes, I did. It was great."

"And it's beautiful. And you know so many people there. So many good friends."

"That's absolutely true too. It's just . . . oh, Christ. It's so hard to explain. I just couldn't."

"But I want to be in Connecticut. Surrounded by my friends. The people who knew Mike."

"Mom, I couldn't. I couldn't go back to Connecticut. I'd go crazy if I did, and I wouldn't be able to take care of you or myself."

"Why?"

"I'd feel . . . like a total failure. Like I never got anywhere. Old. Sad. Trapped."

"Well, I don't understand."

"Don't understand what?"

"Why don't you come back to Connecticut to live?"

A good question. One I was asking myself all the time now.

Why, indeed?

CHAPTER SIX

The Big Bang

There once was a girl and her name was El
Lived at the bottom of a dirty old well
Never learned to write, never learned to spell
What was her name?
Dirty old El.

There once was a boy and his name was Tommy
Lived in a hut like a dirty old swami
Never ate popcorn, only ate salami
What was his name?
Dirty old Tommy.

There once was a girl and her name was Mary
Lived at the bottom of a dirty old . . .

My mother, at the wheel of the car, paused and looked up into the rearview mirror, waiting for my brother and me in the backseat to finish the rhyme.

"Dairy!" We both yelled. I was maybe three, my brother five.

"Never brushed her teeth . . ." my mother offered, and waited again.

"And her arms were hairy!" Tommy said.

"And her face was scary!" I said.

"What was her name?" my mother said.

"Dirty old Mary!" Tommy and I said. And we laughed and laughed.

"Okay," said my mother. "Who's next?"

"Grandma!" said Tommy.

"All right," said my mother. "There once was a girl and her name was Carol . . ."

"Lived at the bottom of a dirty old barrel!"

And so on. No one was exempt. It was our favorite game while the three of us whizzed along our twisty turny woodsy Connecticut roads. I liked to watch my mother drive. I was really interested in the details. The mysterious mechanics, the fantastic skill of coordination, her feet—sandalled and red-toenailed if it was summer—moving from this pedal to that while her hands steered and moved the gearshift and she talked and laughed. How did she do it?

I liked it when she lit one of her unfiltered Kools in the car. I thought the aroma of the first puff of smoke was delicious. Her breath was intoxicating: menthol, minty chewing gum, lipstick. She wore her hair like Lauren Bacall. It was silky, wavy, shiny chestnut brown. She had a little gap between her two front teeth. And you know what they say about people with gaps between their front teeth: sensualists.

We sang in the car, too: "Be kind to your web-footed friends! For this duck may be somebody's mother-r-r-r!" She knew all these woodsy roads by heart. She'd been coming here in the summer from Columbus, Ohio, with her mother and father and older sister since childhood. Her father was a banker and an engineer with a German last name. She told us once that the only effect the Great Depression had on her household in Columbus was that they drove one car instead of two, and the house-keeper gave a lot of food to raggedy men who came to the kitchen door.

Her sister, Caroline, nine years older, was arty and rebellious, and in the 1930s went off to the U.S.S.R. with her boyfriend, Elliot Janeway, who in later years would become a well-known economist. The young couple were ardent socialists. They were going to live the dream. My grandfather the Republican banker and Roosevelt-hater was obliged to keep firing off checks to American Express offices all over Europe to finance the dream, which fell apart in a year or two.

Somewhere in there my mother's parents divorced and my mother moved to New York with my grandmother. I don't think much of my grandfather's money went with them, but my well-born grandmother had some money of her own. Nothing lavish, but a sufficiency. They had a little apartment on Gramercy Park. My mother went to Barnard, dropped out in her sophomore year when she was nineteen and went to work for the *New York Journal-American*. She said when she went to the *Journal-American* building the first time, hoping to get a job, she had no idea who to talk to. It was the doorman who tipped her off: "Go ask for so-and-so on the sixth floor, little lady," he said.

So-and-so on the sixth floor hired her on the spot. That's what you did in 1941 when a long-legged Barnard beauty walked into your office saying she wanted a job. I picture a Damon Runyon sort of scene: He was a man in his forties, and I see him leaning back in his squeaky office chair, wearing a green visor, rubber bands holding his shirtsleeves in place, his arms up and his fingers casually interlaced behind his head while she sits down, crosses her legs and lights a cigarette. Mmmm-hmmm, he thinks.

She started as a copy boy, but went quickly from that to junior reporter and model. Model for the *Journal-American,* that is. I remember being very young, maybe five or six, snooping around in a box in the basement and finding some mysterious big glossy photos. In one, my mother is on a park bench with a sailor. He's looking away from her with a grumpy expression, his hat pushed forward a little for emphasis, one elbow slung up on the armrest of the bench, his other arm resting slouchily on his own leg. She's leaning up against him, holding his arm with both her gloved hands, gazing at him imploringly. Her hair is swept up onto her head and there's a flower pinned to it. Her whole body is slanted toward him in a long graceful diagonal, her traffic-stopping silk-stockinged legs crossed. It's a black-and-white picture, but you know her mouth is red, red. In another picture, my mother and several other women sit at a table in a pleasant little apartment. They're playing cards. There are drinks on the table. A man in a suit, who obviously just came through the door and found the card party, holds a bag of groceries. My mother, cards and cigarette in one hand, points bossily with the other toward the refrigerator.

When I first saw these photos, I thought they were actual scenes from my mother's exotic unknown life before I was born. I was too young to understand that they were carefully staged pictures, shot and used as illustrations for feature articles in the *Journal-American:* "Can a Girl Propose?" Evidently not, or he might get surly on a park bench while she pleads. And "Ladies: Don't Make A House-Husband Out Of Your Man" is certainly a piece of advice every bit as worthy of consideration now as it was then.

She and the forty-something editor who hired her were an item for a while. He squired her around New York, took her to nightclubs, dances, bars. I try to visualize the guy. Married? I have no idea. Possibly. That wouldn't have bothered my mother. If he was, no doubt his wife noticed the extra care and attention he gave to combing his hair, making sure his chin was smooth and putting a fresh hanky in his breast pocket. I can see him looking in the mirror, whistling a little tune, patting after-shave on his face: You lucky devil, you.

The *Journal-American* held a beauty contest at the Stork Club. It was a nifty publicity stunt; the judge was Frank Sinatra. Guess who he picked as the winner?

Sometime very soon after the war ended, she met my father at a Columbia party. My father was a grad, his field English Literature with a specialty in the Arthurian legend. He was fresh from his duties as captain of a Coast Guard corvette doing convoy escort service in the North Atlantic during the last part of the war, protecting troop ships from German U-Boats. He was an expert, self-taught navigator, could chart a course in stormy seas and steer his ship into port, but was city-born and -bred and didn't know how to drive a car until my mother taught him. My mother had been driving since she was thirteen, on those Connecticut roads, without a license and with my grandmother's approval. "Mary's a good little driver," my grandmother would say, and dispatch her to pick someone up at the train or to fetch a bottle of milk at the store.

They got married and moved to Connecticut, to the same town she'd been coming to since she was a child and where she lived until she was seventy-five. They first lived in her family's summer house there. My father took a job teaching English at a local boys' prep school. My brother was born. Then they moved to faculty housing, a little apartment on the campus, and I was born. My brother remembers going back to the first house with Dad to fetch a big brass bell, which had come from Dad's ship and which he'd put up on the garage. Tommy remembers the sailor-braided, shrunk-tight-by-the-North-Sea clanger rope. He has a lot of memories of my parents as a couple, but I have only one: I was sitting on the kitchen counter while my father walked back and forth, back and forth and my mother spoke sharp words to him. I couldn't have been more than two. Curtain descends. When it goes up again, I'm standing in high grass behind a different house. A tall gray three-story house. My mother has left my father, and she and my brother and I are living on two rented floors of the tall gray house.

Miss Janie wore shiny black perforated tie-up shoes. She had skinny little legs, a wren-shaped body, thick glasses magnifying her big watery brown eyes, Brillo hair, a flowered hat and a booming voice. She was Miss Janie to everyone, children and grownups alike.

One beautiful spring day in the early 1950s she took her nursery-school class to the cemetery next door right after a funeral. The family and guests were gone. It was just us and a few guys with shovels. I stood at the edge of the grave with the other little kids, at the very beginning of our lives, looking into the deep hole. The memory is distinct: The grass was brilliant green and the earth was black. Chains clanked as the workers lowered the coffin down, down, down.

What possessed the dotty old bat to impose such a stark lesson in mortality on a bunch of three- and four-year-olds? I can't ask her, because she lies in that same cemetery now, grinning with satisfaction to be there, I'm sure. But I think: Good for you, Miss Janie. Good for you. That was damned ballsy. Watching that box go down was possibly *the* seminal moment of my formative years. Warped me a little, that's for sure; a lurid *memento mori* planted perilously early in my fertile young brain so that I lay awake thinking about eternity and the thud of dirt on coffin lids perhaps more than might be considered wholesome for a child, but worth it. I do believe it was the concentrated fuel-core that jump-started my artistic vision, such as it is, and drives it to this day. Miss Janie helped launch me. I doubt that that's what she had in mind, but she did. For sure, it gave me a head start pondering the Big Picture.

It was also a moment of clear understanding which would stay with me for good: that someday my mother—my mother!—would die. An intolerable idea. I could actually stand the idea of myself dying more readily than I could stand the idea of my mother dying.

Not long after the jaunt to the cemetery, Tommy and I visited my father and he took us to the planetarium in New York. The lights went off and we sat in utter darkness for a few seconds. Then, SPANG! The black heavens lit with stars. A huge amplified voice said: THIS WAS THE NIGHT SKY BEFORE DINOSAURS WALKED THE EARTH.

I let out a wail. I guess I didn't stop, because next thing I knew my father was carrying me out of the planetarium. What scared me? Simple: Infinity. Of time, and of space. I'd grasped it. I understood that if you left the earth and started traveling into space, you would travel forever and ever and ever. I'd already seen an outer-space movie where a guy drifted off into the black universe in his suit and helmet. And I understood that time went on forever too, behind us and in front of us. It was not possible for there to be an end to either time or space, and my wail in the planetarium was a purely primal response to the knowledge, settling in for keeps, that our lives, my mother's included, occur in the territory between the forever out there beyond the stars and that box going down into the ground.

It overwhelmed me. I still don't like it much, but I'm better equipped now to handle it. I know where that tendency to ponder vastnesses came from. That's my father. That's him working in me. It was nature AND nurture: My brother and I rode around twisty turny Connecticut roads with Dad, too, who remarried quickly and lived nearby. We didn't sing and shout in his car, and he never smoked a cigarette in his life, and there was no jolly whizzing along, because he was the most cautious and conscientious driver there ever was, but we had plenty of fun hanging over the back of the seat debating questions he asked us, like: When you drop a stone into a pond and it makes ripples, how far do those ripples travel? Or: If you draw two straight lines right next to each other, and keep drawing them and drawing them, will they ever meet? He wasn't a physicist. He taught English Literature, by then at Columbia. But he *was* a philosopher. And he'd eventually go to England for a year on a Fulbright scholarship to study the Arthurian legend.

By the time I knew him, he'd probably read a couple of thousand books. And he could invent a tale at the drop of a hat. We'd ask him for a Donald Duck story or a story about "our" brontosaurus; he'd say, "Give me a few minutes," and we'd be very quiet while he drove and thought for maybe five or ten miles. Then he'd say, "Okay," and tell a perfectly plotted, suspenseful yarn, either about Donald and Scrooge and Huey, Dewey and Louie or about our brontosaurus friend in his dangerous Mesozoic world, escaping from Tyrannosaurus Rex or surviving volcanic eruptions while pterodactyls glided and screeched in the sky.

The marriage to my mother was short, maybe four and a half years, and I missed most of it. "What was it about Dad that first made you like him?" I used to ask my mother long after they were divorced, because I really was curious. I knew something about why they split, but not much about how they got together. "He was really good-looking," she said (true—when I was five, *Life* magazine put Rock Hudson on its cover one issue and I thought it was my father). "Really smart and witty." That's probably exactly what he would have said about her. So a picture emerges: My father, fresh from the war, tall and handsome in his uniform. My mother, the winner of a Sinatra-judged beauty contest. Columbia and Barnard. 6'2", 5'9".

Out of New York, after two children and a few years in the quiet of a small Connecticut town, there was little left but irreconcilable differences. My father was steady, faithful, kind, highly literate. But the dashing uniform was long gone. Now he was rumpled, tweedy, academic, with an unkempt mat of Black Irish hair. Politically and socially liberal, like my mother (both of them had voted for Roosevelt; later, they'd both vote for Adlai Stevenson), but personally conservative, he was modest, retiring, self-effacing, drank no more than an occasional beer, didn't party or dance.

Dorothy Parker once wrote, in one of her reviews, about the ". . . terrible slow army of the cautious." I believe my mother came to see my father as part of that terrible slow army. She was a racehorse raring to run. She wanted action. She wanted flash and glamour. She busted out, and as much as I love her, I can't say that she did it kindly. I gather, in fact, that her treatment of him could only be called shabby.

This was the early fifties, but there seems to have been no Eisenhower

Era around our house. My mother was part of a fast crowd. There were trysts and tangled webs that would have made John Cheever blush.

My brother says he recalls some hanky-panky at the faculty housing while Dad was out teaching English to prep-school kids. He remembers Mom and a scion of the local gentry drinking martinis in the middle of the day, and the double doors to Dad's study, where there was a couch, closing decisively in his face. And then a former flame of my mother's from her New York days, Alexis, a Russian artist who had married and come to live in the same Connecticut town, brought his mistress up from the city one weekend. He needed a place to park her discreetly but handily for a few days. His wife, of course, was not to know that he had his girlfriend almost under her nose. The girlfriend, a blue-eyed black-haired knockout art student named Violet, wound up on the couch at my mother and father's little faculty apartment. Now my parents were co-conspirators with Alexis, sheltering this languid beauty, who lay about the house doing her nails, waiting for Alexis to get away from his family and pay attention to her.

He must have kept her waiting just a bit too long, because she went off for a one-night stand that weekend with a local fellow whose eye she caught—none other than the martini-drinking scion, my mother's secret lover. My mother was furious, but she was like a diamond thief whose jewels have been stolen. Probably my father didn't know about the scion, but did he know that Alexis—now a close family friend—and my mother had once been an item? I don't know.

Then we were at the tall gray house, where there were more gentleman callers. There was the scion, who evidently patched it up with my mother, and there was another fellow, who, like the first guy, drove a sports car. He also drank martinis. Between the martinis and the sports cars, these guys merge into a composite in my memory: Slim, good-looking, and evidently with an abundance of free time. But there were in fact two of them. Let's call them Neil and Dave.

Sometime around then, when I was maybe three, we went to Mexico. One of these good-looking fellows was along on this trip. Tommy tells me it was Dave. I recall a small village, the grownups warning me to look out for scorpions, whatever those were, and my mother boiling the milk. I remember being out in a boat on a lake in a lush jungle setting, with Dave at the oars, shirtless and tan, rowing leisurely, while my mother swam alongside in a languid sidestroke. I didn't know much at that age, but I knew Dave was watching my mother's legs in the water, and I sort of understood why.

We were down there, I've since figured out, so my mother could get a quickie divorce from my father. Cuernevaca, says Tommy, the Bohemian divorce mecca. My mother left us on the sidewalk with a Mexican family selling melons while she went into a building, Tommy says, and we squatted out there happily, eating melons, until she came out with her papers. Dave must have thought it was another kind of trip, too, and that he was right at the head of the line, but after Mexico he seems to have been phased out, because next thing I remember we were in southern California, and Neil was back in the picture. And he had his sports car—a Jaguar—with him. This can only mean that he drove all the way to California in pursuit of my mother. Imagine that trip: No interstate yet; still a fairly wild and woolly crossing. He probably took Route 66, throttle out all the way, flying on high-octane anticipation. My father appeared briefly, too, trying to win her back—in vain, in vain.

Where and how did she meet Tim Durant? I'll never know, because my mother's memory is shot and Durant is dead. Twenty-two years her senior but slim and handsome à la Neil and Dave, he had a house in Beverly Hills with a big iron gate and a swimming pool. I remember some question as to which one my mother should marry—Neil or Durant—and Neil threatening to drive his Jag off a cliff into the Pacific if she didn't marry him. My brother and I voted for Durant because he had a swimming pool. I hope that wasn't the deciding factor, but she chose Durant. Maybe she liked the sound of the name she got: *Mary Durant*. Neil didn't drive his car off a cliff, but he did, as far as we know, drive it back to Connecticut. He was rushing back to do battle for the hand of another fair damsel: Violet, the gorgeous black-haired art student. But he was fated to lose out again.

My father left on an airplane. His bitterness would be quickly assuaged. He'd be married within a year—to Violet, whom he'd met for the first time when she slept on the couch at his school apartment when she was the secret mistress of my mother's ex-lover and the one-night fling of the guy with whom my mother was cuckolding him.

Tim Durant's name is in the index of Kenneth Anger's *Hollywood Babylon.* It's a small entry, but a seminal one, at the beginning of an account of one of Charlie Chaplin's paternity suit trials. It talks about a young woman, one of thousands in Hollywood hoping to crash the movies, winding up at a party at John Paul Getty's estate in Mexico, where she met an agent for United Artists who then introduced her to Chaplin. That agent was Tim Durant. This was around 1942, when my mother would have been nineteen or twenty, working for the *Journal-American,* gallivanting around New York and winning beauty contests. Durant was forty-two, hobnobbing with oil millionaires on the West Coast and changing the course of world-famous movie directors' lives. Apparently Chaplin didn't hold anything against Durant for that fateful introduction, because they stayed friends. My mother would eventually be introduced to Chaplin by Durant, too.

And she'd eventually marry Durant, at John Huston's place, and bring him to Connecticut to live. And about a year after that Durant would buy the tall, three-story gray house where we'd lived for a while as renters when my mother first left my father. She'd fix it up and live there for the next forty-three years, nineteen of them with Mike.

Why didn't we stay in Beverly Hills and live in Durant's house with the swimming pool? We know that men had a tendency to travel from one coast to another to win my mother's favor. I guess Durant was no exception. Connecticut was where she wanted to live, so that's where we went. In the meantime, he rented his Beverly Hills house to José Ferrer and Rosemary Clooney.

Somewhere right close by is a parallel universe where my mother married Neil. And another where she married Dave (lived at the bottom of a dirty old cave; never took a bath, never took a shave). I'd like to take a peek into both. I realize that in those alternate realities I probably wouldn't be sitting here writing this book, and that possibly my hair would be green and Bruce Willis would be the president of France, but I can't help wondering what else would be different. Chaplin wasn't the only one whose life was changed forever by Tim Durant.

CHAPTER SEVEN

Wicked, Wicked Ways

Above all other things, it is the intensity of his brown eyes, set deep under the supra-orbital ridge. Bent's eyes are incandescent with minute-to-minute humors: tragedy or wit, depression or elation. (Blood, phlegm, choler, black bile.)

He is all in the image of the romantic literary tradition. He is part rogue, part hungry poet, and part matinée idol. And charlatan all the way through, dear love, and still necessary to me. I am susceptible to style rather than content . . .

—*From* QUARTET IN FAREWELL TIME *by Mary Durant*

The classic 1950s science fiction movie *The Day the Earth Stood Still* starred the actor Michael Rennie. Tim Durant looked enough like Rennie to be his long-lost brother—the same handsome sculpted head and abundant silver hair.

Durant was in a couple of movies himself, walk-on (or in one case, ride-on) bit parts in films by his director pals Huston and Ferrer. He did it strictly for fun and for the hell of it. In Ferrer's *Return to Peyton Place,* he plays an acerbic old Yankee in a plaid hunting hat delivering a few pungent lines at a town meeting. He has a look on his face utterly familiar to me and to anyone else who knew him, a smirky satisfaction at delivering a good joke with great skill. And in Huston's *The List of*

Adrian Messenger, he's on a horse in a brief scene, speaking a few lines, then wheeling the horse around expertly and cantering off.

He was the real thing when it came to horses. A 1967 issue of *Life* magazine ran a feature story called "The Galloping Granddad," about him riding in the Grand National Steeplechase at age sixty-seven.

My mother knew how to ride before she met Durant, but bloomed as an equestrienne under his watch. They made the fox-hunting scene in a big way, riding together, traveling around New England and New York State. This probably had a lot to do with Durant giving a try to life in Connecticut. He'd actually been born there himself, went to prep school at Choate and on to Yale. I'd like to know the details of how he migrated west and became a biggish wheel in Hollywood, but that story is lost in the mists of time. So he came back to Connecticut when he took up with my mother, but kept the place in Beverly Hills. Thinking ahead, I'm sure.

He bought my mother a hunter. The horse's official name had been Flying Banner, but my mother thought that was ridiculous and renamed her Birdie. A spectacular photograph shows my mother on Birdie: The shot was taken mid-jump, over a stone wall, probably 1956. She's wearing boots, blazer, jodhpurs, riding hat. She's leaning forward over the reins, her body raised up out of the saddle at the apex of the jump. The horse's ears are pointed forward exuberantly. My mother and the horse are one at that moment, flowing over that stone wall in a great leap of grace and power. Another picture, probably taken on the same day: my mother, looking like a fashion model in her riding clothes, standing in profile at the horse's head, holding the bridle. The horse's ears are forward in this picture, too. My mother and Birdie are looking each other right in the eye, with an attitude of mutual joy and pleasure, even love.

But Durant was a bad, bad influence on my mother. Certain propensities of his matched up a little too well with specific weaknesses of hers. The results were not good—for her, and especially for my brother and me. She'd wanted flash and glamour, and she got it in abundance with Durant. A little too much, in fact. Fox-hunting around New England and environs was fine and dandy, and played a big part in stoking his image of himself as a member in good standing of the ruling class, but he wanted to make the international scene, too. Dublin, London, Paris.

And he wanted his gorgeous, witty young wife on his arm. His wife—not his wife and her two kids. And she let him talk her into it.

Things got off to a bad start before they were even married. A woman friend of my mother's had a sprawling house in rural New York State called "Saloma" where her arty intellectual pals convened. We'd go there for weekends with my mother; the grownups would talk and laugh and drink late into the night. My father, now remarried, had a teaching job in another New York State town close by. One late summer weekend while my brother and mother and I were at Saloma—I was almost five, my brother seven—and Durant was due to appear momentarily, my father came and took us kids out for the day. When he brought us back in the evening, he learned that Durant had come while we were out and that he and my mother were gone. Not gone for dinner or for the weekend. Really gone. To Europe. For the winter.

Dad had no choice but to take us in, immediately, that very day, without a chance to consult his new wife, without any plan or arrangements, the whole thing sprung on him without any warning. A dirty trick, and typical Durant. And my mother went along with it. That's what I mean by a bad influence. He encouraged a side of her that was frivolous, irresponsible, heedless. She was completely under his spell. I can picture them piling her bags into his car, tires squealing and gravel flying as they made their getaway, laughing uproariously at the thought of my father's expression when he came back and found them gone. A joke. A big joke. I wonder how far in advance this caper was planned.

It laid the groundwork for a lot of heartache. We spent that entire winter with my father and stepmother. I was in kindergarten and my brother was in the second grade. My stepmother, Violet, treated us really well, considering, but she was bitter enough about the incident that she never allowed my father to take us in again for anything more than one night. And my father, pussywhipped all the way, could not oppose her.

My mother was gone altogether too often for the four or five years of the marriage to Durant. Too often, and for too long. They went on extended trips, and farmed us out with friends since we couldn't stay with my father. The people we stayed with were always good people, and it was always right there in our town where everything was familiar and we had our friends and our school. We were treated kindly and often had fun, but that didn't prevent us from pining for her keenly. It was a visceral sort of longing, like missing a lover. I remember smelling her tweed jacket once (cologne, menthol) when I was about six and she and Durant had returned from some trip but were about to go away again. I almost fainted with wanting her.

I wonder how those arrangements were made. No doubt Durant paid the people who took us in. There's a dark family rumor that he tried to talk my mother into giving us up for adoption. I don't know if it's true, but I wouldn't put it past him. In any case, she didn't. He had power over her, but not quite that much. And when the first blush was gone and the Durant spell began to lift, I know she deeply regretted letting him take her away from us so much.

The funny thing was that I liked him. It was my brother who got the short end of that stick. Durant treated him badly, psychologically bullying him, insulting and belittling him, calling him a mama's boy—some kind of ludicrous puerile jealousy thing, always when my mother wasn't looking. But sometimes he made her complicit by disguising it as "fun"—like the Christmas when he gift-wrapped banana peels, egg shells, and steak bones and filled my brother's stocking with them, complete with bows and ribbons. My stocking had real gifts in it. What could they have been thinking?

He may have been a coldhearted prick, but he was smart as a whip and had a great sense of humor, a sharp appreciation of the absurd. I remember him laughing until the tears stood in his eyes. He liked practical jokes, especially the kind that verged on the cruel, and he liked to swerve toward trees when we were driving, saying let's just give it a little kiss, while my mother shrieked and laughed, begged him to stop it and clutched at his arm in terror and I jumped up and down in the backseat.

But he was a son of a bitch. Let us not forget that. One afternoon in 1957 or so, my brother and I were out with my father in his car. Dad stopped at the drugstore and happened to run into Durant, who proceeded to have words with my father, and then shove him, right there on the sidewalk in full view of us and anybody passing. In a small town, no less, where everyone knew everyone else. My father, wisely, did not

shove back. He was twenty years younger and big and strong, had a temper himself, could easily have decked Durant—but he had the self-
restraint not to. And my father explained calmly to my brother and me
what Durant was trying to do: provoke my father into hitting him. Ah,
the mysterious world of adults . . .

Adversity, as we know, can be a potent breeding ground, and one of
the things that can grow out of it is art. My mother had known since
college that she was a talented writer. It wasn't just great legs that pro-
pelled her from copy boy to reporter at the *Journal-American* within a
month of being hired. She'd written some short stories, and especially
through the Durant years, kept journals, some of them the secret ones
hidden along with the collection of letters in that box under her bed.

When I was about twelve, I started to sneak the box out when she
was gone and read with my eyes ready to fall out of my head. What I saw
was better than *Lady Chatterley's Lover,* which I would soon read as well.

She used a shorthand of her own devising in her erotic journals. I
caught on quickly, in a nascent sort of way, to the arcane and highly
explicit subject matter, like a budding nuclear physicist reading about
particle theory for the first time. I believe the shorthand was partly
designed to make the material less than instantly accessible and partly a
manifestation of urgency. There was a rushing-toward-climax quality to
the writing that got me seriously hot and bothered while I read, furtive,
one ear tuned for the sound of her car, her footsteps.

The letters, saved over the years, were from various guys, Neil among
them. He was a pretty good writer himself; his letters were particularly
throbbing. Between the letters and my mother's journals, her Byzantine
love life was pretty well covered. I remembered all the guys. And a couple of them were surprises to me. I'd think: *Him?* Jeez! Then I'd think:
Well—hmmm. Yeah. I guess I can see it. And one of them—oh, shocking!—had been a student at the prep-school where my father taught. A
big hulking precocious guy, fulfilling every school kid's wet dream. Did
he first nail her while he was still a student? That part wasn't clear. But
the rest of it was more than clear.

I learned a lot from the contents of that box. One of the things I
learned was that Durant was pretty much a dud in the sack. Probably

this hadn't been so evident in the beginning of their affair, what with the excitement of the globetrotting, the illustrious company he kept and all the rest of it. But he wasn't a giver. Not in the ways that my mother yearned for. I remembered her cry: *You don't want me. You don't need me!*

A couple of years into their union, she went to a psychiatrist. She wanted to find out why she had married such a distant loveless man. Those were the days of classic Freudian analysis. What she found out— surprise!!—was that she had married a guy just like her father. But the psychiatrist, apparently, was intrigued. He wanted to see for himself. He asked for a session alone with Tim Durant.

God knows how my mother talked him into it; probably he went with the attitude that he'd straighten out this psychiatrist fellow and all this damned analysis nonsense once and for all. He and the psychiatrist spent an hour together. Whatever words were spoken between the two of course we will never know, but the shrink's words to my mother afterward ring clear down through the decades. He called Tim Durant (and this is an exact quote) a "psychiatric monument," and said to her: I don't usually tell my patients this, but my advice is to get as far away from that man as you possibly can. Immediately.

I have to give Durant credit, though. When the marriage lay broken on the rocks, and she'd taken up with various men, and he split permanently back to Beverly Hills, he wasn't in the least vindictive. He left her the house, in her name and all paid for. The tall gray house.

And he proved himself a good sport in other ways. I saw him once, years and years later, in the mid 1970s. I dropped in unannounced at his messy little apartment in Santa Monica (the Beverly Hills house was long gone). He was glad to see me. There I was, grown up, in my twenties. We talked about a lot of things.

One of the things we talked about was her first novel, and specifically, her brilliantly drawn and unflattering portrait of him as Hoyt Bentley. A lot of people would have been bitter, but he wasn't.

After the split with Durant, my mother's frivolous era began to come to a close. She worked hard to make things up to my brother and me. She took us on a great trip to Ireland in the summer of '59. We met Huston, with whom she'd stayed friends, met his kids, who were close to our age, and played all over his estate where she'd married Durant. Two of her lovers rendezvoused with her in Ireland (not at the same time). This was perfectly okay with us; they were both nice guys and God knows we'd been raised not to be uptight about sex (for which I'm eternally grateful to my mother; the "sexual revolution" of the sixties and seventies was no big deal to me). Tommy and I had a ball, exploring ruins and soaking up the haunted atmosphere of Ireland. And she started to seriously address her writing.

Her affairs, steamy and numerous though they were, did not result in anything permanent or deeply satisfying. There was a lot of frustration, but she poured her energy into her work.

Her first novel came out in early 1963 to ecstatic reviews. Said one: "Mary Durant is obviously meant to write about the nuances of human attraction and repulsion. She does a delicate and frightening job. First novels of this discipline, assurance and beauty of detail are altogether rare."

She did a delicate and frightening job on Durant, and on other people, too. The central character is based on a woman with whom my mother had been friends for years until a serious falling-out. The woman was a seductive, scheming taker, and in her novel my mother creates a merciless holographic portrait of her anti-heroine by telling the story from the first-person points of view of four of the woman's "victims." The lives of these four are interlocked, too, whether they know it or not, through their association with the woman.

All but one of the major characters in the novel were based on real people, one of them my mother herself. When I read it, a light bulb went on in my head. Since I knew well the people from whom the characters were fashioned, I could see what was real and what was my mother's invention and innovation, and grasped instantly the Dr. Frankensteinian process of synthesis by which a fiction writer uses truth and invention to create characters and breathe life into them. It was an invaluable shortcut to understanding, a veritable crash course in writing. My mother had already put such authors as John Cheever, Flannery O'Connor, Mary McCarthy and Brian Moore under my nose, and I, a precocious little reader, had dug their work, even if I didn't grasp 100 percent of what I was reading. Now, directly because of my mother's work, I was initiated somewhat into the mystery of how they did what they did—and why.

Durant may have been a good sport about his deconstruction at my mother's hands, but not everyone else was. The woman on whom the female protagonist was based recognized herself and tried—unsuccessfully—to sue my mother. Several other women, including my mother's own sister, flattered themselves that they were the ones my mother had written about, and vied for the privilege of being outraged. My mother thoroughly enjoyed the whole experience.

My mother made Hoyt Bentley's eyes dark brown. Durant's eyes were in fact blue. She also reversed an important dynamic between herself and him. In the novel, Jane Bentley (the character based on my mother) is rich and holds the purse strings while Bent (his nickname throughout the book) is dependent on her, but always wheedles out of her what he wants. Durant, while he was not exactly wealthy, had some bucks and was the one who paid the bills when he was married to my mother. These variations on the truth ultimately enrich the truth. Making Bent's eyes dark was an efficient way of darkening his character. Making Jane the one with the money, forever financing this or that whim or fancy of her husband's because she could not resist him, adroitly illustrated the emotionally manipulative way Durant ran the show.

While Bentley-Durant doesn't emerge exactly unscathed from the pages of her novel, my mother took care to round him out. He actually gets a few strokes of insightful sympathy, and we get a glimpse into his obscure soul. There's a paragraph toward the end where he runs into his now ex-wife and her friends at a gallery opening. He watches them, thinking how confident, assured and safe they all are in each other's company, and reflects poignantly:

> . . . I looked at the circle of faces and felt the old pangs of exclusion. I would never be included. I would never catch up with them. There would never be any softness or concern for me. I would always be the indiscernible figure in the small end of the glass . . .

At the end of my visit with Durant in Santa Monica, the last time I ever saw him, he said to me, "Tell your mother I'm glad I was able to contribute something to her life."

★ ★ ★

At another point in the novel, Jane writes in her journal:

> *No one says what I want to hear: "You are tired, let me help*
> *you. You are sad, let me make you laugh. You are lonely, let me*
> *keep you company . . . "*

These lines sum up the deficiencies of my mother's marriage to
Durant and of her many liaisons that followed, until she found Mike. I
know the words are my mother's own, thoroughly hers, unfiltered
through the medium of fiction.

CHAPTER EIGHT

Our Town

I want to go home.

When my mother and Durant were in California, he surely heard those words from her, a lot, just as I did. When she spoke them to her new husband, he was unable to resist. She was at the height of her persuasiveness, her life in front of her, and the words had power. When she spoke them to me, she was broken, old, diminished and pleading, but the words were no less powerful. Not enough to make me go back, but enough to evoke "home" so vividly that there were times when it seemed as if the ancient melancholia, not content to lie in wait, had uncoiled itself, left its lair, searched me out and found me at the other end of the continent. And it made me understand the extent to which we'd cut out her heart by taking her away from there. The town was my mother, and my mother was the town. Whatever I am, that place made me. And my mother made me.

Yes, life would have been very different indeed if we'd stayed in Beverly Hills. I don't think Tim Durant and Miss Janie ever met; if they had, she would have been the object of his considerable derision, and she'd have loathed him in return. But the two of them were close partners in helping to create the mysterious, complicated push-me-pull-you force field that emanates from the town, that haunts my brother and me to this day. Not that my wicked stepfather and my batty old nursery-

school teacher did it all by themselves, but they were major players. I like
to picture them riding in a car together for all eternity in a sort of existential Driving Miss Janie, Durant at the wheel swerving toward trees
while she whacks him with her cane . . .

In that same cemetery where Miss Janie took us, and not far from where
she's in repose, there's a tree with letters carved on it. That tree is a perfect cemetery tree. It has smooth bark, a big sturdy immortal-looking
trunk and long lush droopy branches with whispery, rustling leaves. You
have to know what the carved letters are in order to recognize them.
Forty years have made them spread and bloom into illegibility. I know
what they are, though: "T.C. + A.C." My brother and his best friend,
André Chernov. The old guy who tended the cemetery was furious
with Tommy and André, and called the parents. André got into some
trouble, but my mother just laughed. "So they carved their initials in a
tree," she said. "Big deal. It's what kids do."

We've known André from birth. His father was my mother's erst-
while flame Alexis, the very same Alexis who stashed his illicit New York
girlfriend with my parents one long-ago weekend. My parents divorced,
but Alexis and his wife did not, and the Chernovs were our tightest family friends. Alexis was a classically trained artist whose gift put you in
mind of Rembrandt or Michelangelo. His family left Russia just before
the revolution and moved to Germany. He was the same age as the century, and in the 1920s went to live in Berlin. There he was, a brilliant
educated young man in the prime of his prime, an artist, handsome and
black-eyed, in the heart of the Bertolt Brechtian cultural hub of Europe
between the great wars.

As strong young men do, he worked at different jobs. One was in a
foundry. When we were little kids, and Alexis was in his fifties, he'd take
off his shirt and solemnly show us the scars on his back from flying bits
of molten metal. He was also tacitly showing us his ropy, powerful
physique. Another of his jobs had been as a court artist. He'd been
there for the trial of Fritz Haarman, a pervert and mass murderer extra-
ordinaire whose shenanigans make Jeff Dahmer look like a dilettante.

Once in the 1970s Alexis pulled a couple of sketches from a portfolio and showed them to me. The first was of Haarmen in the courtroom during the trial; the other was Haarmen just a few moments before his execution by decapitation. Alexis was a portrait artist without peer. When he showed me those sketches, fifty years fell away in an instant and I was looking right into the colorless amoral eyes of the Butcher of Hanover.

And what, you might ask, of the wife behind whose back Alexis was sneaking around, the mother of his only child? Katrina Chernov was one of the great madwomen of all time. If ever there was someone who was not a member of Dorothy Parker's terrible slow army, it was Katrina. To call her merely "mad" would be to do her a great disservice. Mad she was, but she was also the living antidote to everything humdrum, tepid, quotidian. Infuriating, too, of course—able to exasperate you to the point of spluttering incredulousness, eventually eighty-sixed from several people's houses and lives, including my mother's, but never, ever ordinary, and often on fire with inspiration. Today, they'd call her bipolar. Back then, the name was manic depression. She and my mother were pals for years until their final falling-out.

Clinically, Katrina was a textbook case. She went from dizzy highs to the blackest lows on a cycle as regular and predictable as the movements of the stars, with stages in between where she was either on her way up or on her way down. The time from her highest point to her lowest was about two months. Every year, year in, year out, as long as she lived. She was about fifteen years older than my mother, but you would never have known it. She seemed immune to age. Her skin stayed smooth, her body limber. My mother had a theory: The time Katrina spent in the "down" (as my mother called it) part of her manic cycle was a form of suspended animation. All processes slowed, including the process of age. My mother may have been on to something. Katrina lived to almost ninety, and her honey-brown hair never turned gray.

When she was "down," she became a ghost. She retreated to her room, drew the curtains, rarely left her big four-poster bed where she'd watch her black-and-white rabbit-eared TV all day and all night. She occasionally cracked the door just enough to whisper to her son. If she dressed, it was in black, and she wore her hair in a severe knot.

Gradually, she would emerge from this chrysalis of gloom. When I say emerge, I mean emerge. Two months later might find her scampering barefoot across the village green in a milkmaid outfit, hair streaming, shoulders bare, eyes blazing. When she was "up," we kids thought she was the most fun grownup around. None of the other mothers, not even mine, let you ride on the luggage rack on the roof of the car under the full moon at sixty miles an hour on country roads in the middle of the night.

The Chernovs lived in what had once been the stable and carriage-barn of a defunct grand estate. Built in the 1860s and converted to a house sometime in the early 1940s, it was big, dark, sprawling. A rickety crooked wooden staircase led up to what had once been the hayloft, then Alexis's studio. Downstairs, at the other end of the enormous main room where horses and carriages once rolled in, a heavy door led to another wing of the house and Katrina's and André's bedrooms and the one tiny bathroom.

The Chernov house was done in a style I'd call Fallen Baronial. It was (still is) magnificent, in an entropic, old-world sort of way. A long, refectory-type dining table with ten tall carved gothic chairs and stately candlesticks. A fireplace at one end of the main room big enough to burn tree-trunks, an ancient dark velvet couch and a couple of tattered-but-noble stuffed chairs arranged in front of it. At the other end of the huge room, an antique grand piano, untuned for decades and with half the keys stuck. Shelves packed with dusty leather-bound nineteenth-century German-language books. A display of bones from the horse cemetery out back. A threadbare hotel-lobby-sized Oriental carpet on the floor and heavy dark tasseled drapes. A horse-drawn sleigh from the eighteen-nineties. The only window in the main room, which was all old dark unpainted wood, was a bay window where the big sliding stable doors had once been, so even on the brightest summer day the house was brooding, shadowy, cool. In the winter radiators hissed and clanked inadequately here and there, and it was often necessary to wear an overcoat inside the house. Alexis's paintings and sketches, some of heroic proportions with biblical themes, looked down from the walls. Alexis liked to thump the ceiling over the long table occasionally with a broom handle, dislodging ancient bits of hay, to show that he lived in a stable.

There had once been money, but it was mostly gone by the 1950s. Alexis supported the household doing commercial art. He was never paid what he was worth, so it was a life of genteel poverty, always on the brink by the time I, my brother and André were little kids running around that house, one of the first places I saw, its molecules and ambience some of the first I breathed when I opened my eyes on this world. It was quite literally a second home to me and my brother.

To get from our house to the Chernov's you could follow the roads, or, if you were fast and agile like us, you could take the shortcut: Up the hill, through the woods and the cemetery got you there in about eight minutes.

About a hundred paces from Miss Janie's final resting place is a modest flat stone, flush with the clipped green grass. It reads: *Lydia Wood, 1905–1962.*

My piano teacher. A maiden lady, Miss Wood lived with her impossibly ancient parents and her younger brother. For five years my mother dropped me off at Miss Wood's house once a week, where I was always sent into the kitchen to wash my paws before I was allowed to touch the gorgeous gleaming black grand piano in her parlor. For five years I resolutely resisted learning to read music, and she kindly and just as resolutely persisted in trying to teach me. I know I drove her to despair, because I was not in fact totally devoid of musical ability. I played fairly well, but always by ear, which of course limited me to just a few pieces.

Too bad I was so damned stubborn. It wasn't that my mother was trying to make me into a concert pianist or anything like that. My mother was a big believer in *fun,* and she was simply trying to add a skill to my repertoire that would help make my grownup life as much fun as it could possibly be. People who are able to sit down and play the piano can open just about any door in the world, she said, and she was right. So I spent many, many hours, many years, on the bench next to Miss Wood. I may not have been learning to read music, but I was my mother's daughter, and I was alert.

I remember Miss Wood's silver hair pulled back into a spinster's bun. But I also remember her soft fuzzy low-necked short-sleeved sweaters and pearl necklaces, her smooth pale skin, her voluptuous bosom, her lavender aroma, her slim tailored wool skirts with the zippers up the back, her silkily stockinged legs, her suede high heels working the pedals. When she went out, she wore a flowing overcoat, a beret and a long elegant matching scarf. And I remember the younger brother. The much younger brother.

He was a grownup, who wore a hat and had a job and drove a car, but even I, aged six when I first saw him, thought in an inchoate way that those bent, creaky gray people I occasionally encountered back in the kitchen were sort of old to be his parents . . .

That's right. After Miss Wood's early death from a cerebral hemorrhage, which I hope had nothing to do with pupils who refused to learn, the story made its inevitable way out into the world: He wasn't her brother. He was her son. Her parents, those plain country folk moving diffidently in the background, had conspired to protect her in a crisis, probably sometime in the early 1930s. Did the son know all along? I could ask him. He still lives in that house.

Ah. Grown sons living with their mothers. We had a lot of those odd couples in our town. Not quite the same arrangement as Miss Wood and her boy. Most of them were elderly widowed mothers and their never-married middle-aged sons. They functioned exactly as couples in many ways: Son driving Mama to the movies, escorting her to the Firemen's Carnival or the theater or to a town meeting, taking her shopping. And these bachelor fellows were not bums mooching off their mothers. They were not lying around the basement playing the guitar. Like husbands, they went off to work every day—as insurance salesmen, lawyers, teachers. Probably Mama cooked, though I suspect that some of these husband-sons had to tie on aprons when they got home in the evening.

My mother had a wicked fantasy: She said she'd like to give a dinner party and invite all of the town's mother-son couples. She pictured them sitting at the table, the realization of what they all had in common dawning on them one by one.

Bill and Ellen Wilcox were such a pair. Ellen was a fiercely intelligent old lady with a house full of books, a string of degrees and a prolific pen. She and my mother were good friends. When my mother went to New York to work as an editor a few years after she split with Durant, Ellen wrote to her three or four times a week. My mother kept all those letters—witty, biting, erudite observations of the big world and small-town life—which eventually amounted to hundreds. "There's a book in this," my mother said. I remember her reading a favorite opening line from one of Ellen's letters:

> "Mary, my dear—The weather has turned, and today it rains on the just and the unjust . . ."

"The just and the unjust! I *love* it!" my mother exclaimed, then put her head back and laughed with pure delight. When someone died, Ellen would say archly of that person: "Well, *his* troubles are over." My mother loved that, too, and it entered her lexicon.

Bill, Ellen's only child, was a big, easygoing slobby guy, about six-three and four hundred pounds. He worked as a paint salesman. He drove a big Dodge sedan that sagged almost to the ground on the driver's side. It had a bent antenna, a faded vinyl roof and a sticker on the rear bumper: MASURY PAINT IS GOOD PAINT. If you ran into him in town, and you were in your car, he'd stand and chat with you through the rolled-down window, his enormous stomach right about at your face-level, his bellybutton peeking out of his straining shirt like a third eye. To his mother, he was "Billy." I know she wished for greater things for her Billy than to be a paint salesman in a country town, but she loved him as he was. They lived in a cramped, cluttered old house. Ellen had a stroke and ended up in a wheelchair. When I was a teenager, she hired me to come for a day while Billy was at work. The disorder was getting away from her. Billy wasn't much help in that department. There was a staircase, which of course she couldn't use, and it was stacked all the way up with papers, books, magazines, catalogues, unread mail. She had me go through the piles on every step and she'd decide whether things got tossed or kept.

On the highest step, in a dark dusty corner, I found a stash of *Playboy*s. Don't worry, Billy, I thought, up at the top of the stairs where Ellen couldn't see me pushing them further back into the shadows. Your secret is safe with me. Except of course that I told my mother, who pumped me for details of what I found inside the house. She thought it was hilarious about the *Playboys*. Just you wait, my mother always said. As soon as Ellen dies, Bill will find a wife.

My mother's prediction was wrong, though. After Ellen's death he lived on in the dilapidated house, alone, drove his Dodge sedan to work and back, his *Playboys* providing him with probably the only feminine companionship, aside from his mother's, he'd ever known. *Masury Paint is Good Paint.*

In our town, we had not just one but two expatriate Russians with mad American wives. Alexis's eyes were so black that iris and pupil were indistinguishable; Colonel Boris Samsonoff had eyes as pale as a winter sky in Siberia. The Colonel had been an officer under Tsar Nicholas. Like Alexis, he'd left Russia before the revolution. And like Alexis, whatever money he might have had once was mostly long gone.

He was in his seventies by the time I knew him. My mother had first glimpsed him when she was a teenager. *God,* she said; *he was the handsomest man I ever saw in my life.* You could still see it when he was old. Tall, broad shoulders, a full head of wavy white hair and a Slavic caste to those eyes. He'd been a master Cossack rider in his prime. My mother told us that she remembered him in his younger days riding his horse into town, wearing his old Cossack coat.

He had a few horses. He gave riding lessons to children, and I was one of them. Again, my mother, such a fine rider herself, was simply trying to add something fun to my life. I never learned to jump. It was a little like my recalcitrance with Miss Wood. The Colonel wasn't quite as sweet-natured as Miss Wood about my failings. I remember him red-faced and raging once when I refused to gallop toward the raised bar. I was about eight, but somehow I knew it wasn't really me he was so angry at.

His wife, Margaret, was a painter whom he'd met and married in Paris. I liked her a lot—she was fun and friendly, to kids especially. She wasn't quite as wild as Katrina in the "up" part of her manic cycle, but she did occasionally drive to the post office in her nightgown. The Samsonoffs were not the intimates that the Chernovs were, so I don't know the details of what went on at home, but I don't think it was fun for the Colonel. I suspect great quantities of alcohol were involved.

Young though I was, it often seemed to me that there was a cloud of sadness around him.

He had real Russian soul, though. One day when my mother had dropped me off for a lesson he said solemnly that he had something to show me. We went into the barn, and he held the head of one of the horses tenderly between his two huge hands so that its eye was framed. "Look," he said. "See how beautiful it is." And we stood there and gazed into the depths of the horse's big purply-brown limpid eye with the long black lashes. And he was right. It was beautiful. Like my years on the bench beside Miss Wood, this was not wasted time. And of course, like everything else, I had my mother to thank for it.

The Colonel and Margaret had two sons. The one I knew best was named Ivan, and by the time he was a young man he was at least as handsome as his father had once been. Black hair, blue eyes. A true heart-throb. My mother definitely checked him out. I may have been just a little kid, but I certainly noticed him, too. He was an athlete, a runner, decades before jogging was invented. My mother and I, riding in the car, often caught glimpses of him sprinting along leafy roads around town. My mother would draw her breath in sharply with appreciation, and I'd see her glancing in the rearview mirror for another look after we passed him. And he was a really nice guy with a sunny disposition. Women were mad for him. The Colonel adored him.

Ivan got some kind of bone cancer in his leg. They cut it off, all the way up to his pelvis. He wore an elaborate prosthesis for a while— elaborate because they'd cut off so much that there was no stump at all—and then he died. On the day of Ivan's funeral, the Colonel took his old Cossack rifle and blew his head off. I remember my mother answering the phone and bursting into tears. So much for my riding lessons. And I really, really missed him . . .

A classy, witty educated beauty like my mother moved with ease in elite circles, and my brother and I were beneficiaries. Because of her, we met and got to know all kinds of fascinating people. The artist Alexander Calder lived in our town. Arthur Miller, who still lives there, was his close friend and neighbor, their properties in the rolling hills adjoining one another. My mother knew them both.

Later, when Arthur Miller was married to Marilyn Monroe, my mother was a guest at a dinner at the Calders'. Mr. and Mrs. Miller were supposed to be there too, but they were late, and dinner was held up for one hour, then two. My mother said there were a lot of phone calls back and forth between the two houses. Mr. Miller was having a difficult time getting his wife out the door. Calder was growing impatient. Finally he'd had enough. After perhaps the fourth or fifth phone call, my mother heard Sandy, a down-to-earth guy if ever there was one, say in his growly voice, "Tell Miller if he doesn't get over here in ten minutes he can't borrow my extension ladder anymore!"

Calder's studio was one of my childhood haunts. I watched him make mobiles, wire sculptures, paintings. I was there for a performance of his famous miniature circus. He made a miniature crossbow and arrows to go with it for my brother. The Calder house was a wonderland of arty esoterica and sly humor. The toilet-paper holder in one of the bathrooms was a hand, life-sized, made of heavy copper wire. The roll of paper sat on the vertical extended middle finger. Typical Calder, and something it probably took him about three minutes to make. In the kitchen ornate wiry whisks, giant pasta spoons and whimsical serving forks, all Calder creations, hung from the ceiling over the stove like one of his mobiles, and the atmosphere was redolent with cloves and red wine.

Once, when I was perhaps ten, I was there with my mother. While the grownups talked, I amused myself looking through some of Calder's hundreds of photography books, and I came upon a picture that still rises up in my mind occasionally. It was a close-up of the head of a corpse lying in a coffin after a grave robbery in a New Orleans cemetery. The corpse's gold teeth had been taken. The bottom jaw, unkindly dislocated by the robbers, lay flat on the chest. The face was bloated with putrefaction and the eyes bulged from the sockets. I remember closing the book immediately, stunned, opening it again for another peek, then slamming it shut again. This was the pornography of death. Over the years, whenever I went to their house, I'd wait until no one was looking, find that book and dare myself to look at the picture. That picture might have been as important to my education as the trip to the cemetery with Miss Janie. The hard facts were not softened or hidden or sugar-coated: Death is *real*. Decades later, when death set up house-keeping in my mother's poor brain in the form of Alzheimer's, that photograph would flit through my dreams from time to time.

I'm looking at another picture right now: It's a big black-and-white glossy print. It's obvious that this is the work of a serious pro. No flash was used; the light comes from a tall 1790s-vintage multi-paned window in the background, brilliantly overexposed so that you can barely see what's outside. Three people sit at the end of a long wooden table. There are the remnants of lunch—French bread, a bottle of wine, wooden bowls. Cigarette smoke curls in the air; wisps of steam rise from a big shiny kettle on the stove. One of the three people is a child—me. On either side of me, talking across the table so that they're in semi-profile, are a man and a woman. The silvery window-light picks out their features: The man's brainy-looking forehead and bald pate, thick glasses and bushy mustache, the woman's fantastically handsome nose and tousled dark hair. It's the Calders' kitchen. The man is Saul Steinberg, the woman is my mother, and the picture was taken by Gjon Mili, one of the greats of twentieth-century photography and my mother's lover. No doubt they met in that house. My mother's body language and the way the shot was framed make it plain that they were already doing it when that picture was taken. And of course, I knew. If you look closely at the window, you can see snow on the panes and ghostly bare branches beyond. While my prospects for riding in the Steeplechase and being the life of the party playing sambas on the piano may not have been sterling, plenty else, all thanks to my mother, as always, was sinking in.

Her versatility, for instance. Our town was sociologically complex, and my mother moved with ease and assurance through all the various strata. This made at least as strong an impression on me and my brother—maybe stronger—as all her arty intellectual connections. A guy named Zip Zumph was our plumber for a while. My father, explaining to my brother and me the theoretical system of categorizing people according to their physical types as either endomorphs, mesomorphs or ectomorphs, cited Zip as a perfect example of an endomorph: shortish, thickset, barrel-shaped. He was smart, talkative and funny. After he fixed something in our house, he'd stay for a cup of coffee and he and my mother would shout and laugh. They became pals. She called him "Zipper."

Zip had a wife, but no one ever saw her. After Zip and my mother had been friends for a while, we got an invitation to dinner at the Zumphs'. I don't know where my brother was, but he wasn't there for this expedition. It was just my mother and me. Zip's wife turned out to be a beautifully groomed and coiffed, rather stout Puerto Rican lady who spoke almost no English. The dinner was formal and a wee bit strained. Zip wasn't anywhere near as relaxed as he was at our house. Part of it was a touch of class consciousness creeping in (not because of my mother; she always put everyone at ease), and part of it was that Zip's gracious wife was something of a nut case.

She had no children, but about five hundred dolls that we spent the evening being introduced to by name. My mother exclaimed and complimented like a trooper while Zip grew quiet and reflective. Later, my mother and I tried to imagine Mrs. Zumph's life in a tiny Connecticut town, at home all day every day with her dolls.

Zip was a Swamp Yankee, which you were if your family had been in town for generations and you talked a certain way. The breed is specific to a small part of rural northwestern Connecticut. The term is not a pejorative. It's a label worn with wily pride by members of the tribe, some of whom have been known to cultivate the speech and mannerisms as if they'd formed a Preservation Society. Taciturnity is a must (either that or chatty as all hell, like Zipper), as is an economy of mouth motion (Wumbeer? Translation: Do you want a beer?), the liberal sprinkling of oaths and expletives (Christ, the goddamn car fell through the goddamn fuckin' ice), and especially when you're cracking a joke, the maintenance of a deadpan demeanor. Christ, yeah.

A friend of mine bought himself a very old, very used Alfa Romeo for a few hundred dollars when he was a teenager. He was really excited about it. He took it to the local garage to get it checked out. He'd always known that Wayne, one of the mechanics, looked on him and his friends as snot-nosed hifalutin' types (from "up the hill"). But Wayne didn't say anything. He just glanced at the car, rolled under it for a few minutes, rolled back out, looked at my friend, then punctured his dreams with three little words, delivered with perfect expressionless Swamp Yankee malicious glee (try saying this out loud without moving your lips, in four descending notes, and you'll get a fair approximation): "She's rusted out." My mother and brother and I practiced our Swamp Yankee a lot on each other, around the house, riding in the car.

I went to the local public school through the eighth grade. It certainly would have been possible for my brother and me to be snobs, but with my mother as our example, we weren't. Quality was everything, but her definition of quality had strictly to do with whether or not someone was *interesting*. You could be John Huston or you could be Zip Zumph, and you could be pals with my mother, as long as you did not commit the one sin unforgivable in her eyes: being a bore.

Not that you couldn't fall from grace. Katrina Chernov was certainly a live wire. But like a lot of bipolar people, she had a problem with what they nowadays call "boundaries." That's a polite way of saying that when they're flying high they're apt to, say, barge into your house when you're not there and rearrange the furniture. Once my mother came home from errands in the afternoon and found Katrina upstairs in her bedroom trying on her clothes. Katrina wasn't even slightly embarrassed. Quite the contrary. My mother said she remembered Katrina's mad manic dilated pupils as she swirled the long skirt of an evening dress with a grand fashion-model flourish when she saw my mother coming up the stairs.

But that wasn't what finally made my mother eighty-six Katrina from her house and life. Nor was it the time my mother discovered that someone had stolen some of her clothes. They were just plain gone: a couple of sweaters, a dress, a skirt. Katrina was the prime suspect, and so one afternoon when we knew everyone was away my mother and I went to the Chernov house and snuck into Katrina's bedroom with the huge dusty tapestry and the four-poster bed with the ancient tattered curtains and searched her closets and bureau drawers for the missing clothes. We didn't find a thing. If she took them, she was clever enough to hide them. I personally don't think it was Katrina, though I have no alternate suspects. My mother always thought she did. It remains one of the great unsolved mysteries of the ages.

And my mother didn't break it off with Katrina the time she actually did steal something, right out from under my mother's nose. At some point in the past, before I was born, I think, my mother had stored a few pieces of antique furniture with Katrina, things from her parents' long-ago summer house. The agreement was that Katrina could enjoy them until such time as my mother wanted them back: a mirror, an embroidered footstool, a small table. The pieces were old and dark and right at home in the Chernov milieu. They looked as if they'd been there forever. So much so that when my mother tried to reclaim them, Katrina said, "Mary, dear, you're mistaken. These pieces have been in my family for generations."

No. The end came one rainy afternoon. It was not over clothes or furniture. It was over a box of doughnuts. My brother and André and Katrina had gone to the movies (my mother always instructed us to ride in the backseat, for safety, when we drove with Katrina), bought doughnuts on the way home, and there was some question as to how they should be divvied up. When Katrina burst into my mother's house demanding her share of the doughnuts, my mother reached her limit. Blazing with anger, my mother tossed her out, and I don't think that over the next nearly forty years until Katrina's death they ever exchanged another word.

The split didn't affect my mother's friendship with Alexis. Their friendship would eventually suffer, but much later, and it would have nothing to do with Katrina. It would have to do with my mother's novel (Alexis's old-world vanity was offended, so the story goes, because my mother made him an avuncular friend, not a lover, of the female protagonist). By the time my mother threw Katrina out, Mr. and Mrs. Chernov had been estranged for years, under the same roof, he at one end of the rambling house and Katrina at the other. They met occasionally in the kitchen, I think.

The town had a drama group, and for a few years there was a miraculous convergence of talent resulting in some awesomely good professional-quality theatre. Alexis designed and painted sets. My mother was one of many fine actors and sometimes directed. A close friend of hers, Phil, a brilliant veteran theatre guy, came up from New York to direct shows, staying at our house while he did it. When I was about twelve, they put on Tennessee Williams's *Glass Menagerie* as theatre-in-the-round. My mother played Laura, the sad girl with the limp. I went to every performance, choosing a different vantage each night. I felt magically invisible and voyeuristic. One night, I positioned myself so that I watched through the shelves of glass figurines. Somewhere in the first act, Laura limped to the shelves and took one of the pieces in her hand while she spoke. There was my mother, about four feet away, looking through the glass and the invisible wall right at me, without a flicker. And I understood: At that moment she was not my mother. She was Laura, a crippled spinster girl waiting in vain for a gentleman caller.

My mother did such a convincing job as Laura that it upset some people. They didn't like to see her lame and dejected and tragic. My mother had no patience with this. "Idiots," she said. "What do they want? A steady diet of Gilbert and Sullivan?"

Another production during the theatre's glory days was T.S. Eliot's *Murder in the Cathedral.* It was Phil directing again, and Alexis designing the costumes and the posters, bloodred on black. My mother played the Tempter, a seductive, Puck-like entity tantalizing Thomas à Becket onto the shoals. Tommy played one of the hooded monks who eventually carry the dead archbishop out of the church. (He missed his cue one night because he was out in the bushes with a girlfriend.) I, aged thirteen, was in the chorus, wearing a hooded medieval-style robe, speaking lines like: "*. . . the starved crow sits in the field, attentive, while in the wood the owl rehearses the hollow note of death . . .*" while my mother, in bright tights and gossamer silk, sidled and insinuated and slithered around the doomed archbishop. This time, no set was needed; the show was put on in the local Episcopal church, a magnificent neo-gothic stone structure that really was like a miniature cathedral.

The audience sat in the pews, the reflections of candle flames glinted in the stained glass, a few well-placed theatre lights pierced the gloom so that the actors moved in pools of illumination. It was thrilling. It was such a hit that we actually took the show on the road, putting it on in a real cathedral in nearby Waterbury where it sold out every night.

Not everyone got it. There were a few detractors in our town. One

woman, her mouth pursed with reproval, said she thought it was scan-
dalous to put on a play in a church. Again, my mother was scathing. "If
she weren't such an illiterate blockhead," my mother said about the
woman, "if she knew anything at all about history, she'd know that the tradition of putting on plays in churches started in the Middle Ages as a way
to get the teachings out to the common man." No, my mother didn't suffer bores, and she didn't suffer "dumbbells."

But she had all kinds of friends. Some of her friends were women
and men who drank martinis and laughed too loudly, some were book-
ish, scholarly and prim, some were farmers. And some of my mother's
pals were the offbeat sort that made Tim Durant very uptight indeed
and were, I suspect, one of the banes of their short marriage. Like Kevin
and Jerry.

Kevin and Jerry were in big demand at dances. Wifeless, and superb
hoofers, they whirled the ladies all over the floor, my mother included.
"What DIVINE dancers!" my mother would exclaim, exhilarated, after
a party. They worked in New York, something to do with production
design for TV, and they had a house in the country where they came on
weekends and for the summer. They had fluffy Persian cats and little
yappy dogs. They had white-painted wrought-iron curlicue chairs in
their dining room, lavish flower arrangements in the living room. In the
bedroom they had twin beds with festoons of green silk on the head-
boards and walls. I thought it was really neat that these two guys had this
cool house together. One night when we were there for dinner, and my
mother and Kevin and Jerry were talking, laughing and carrying on,
Tommy, who was maybe thirteen to my eleven and evidently much
more worldly than I, whispered that Kevin and Jerry were "homos."
"Nah!" I said. "Oh, man, it's so obvious," he said. "Hmm," I said, and
gave it some serious thought.

When children contemplate the mysterious lives of grownups, they
must fill in the blanks and learn fast. I had a fair grasp of why the
Colonel blew himself away. But why did George Sondergard kill himself? And why did he do it the way he did?

George owned a prosperous insurance agency in town. He lived in
a fine big white colonial house. He had a wife and kids. He acted in

plays, a couple of times with my mother, and he sang really well—I remember him in a musical she directed. He was a cheerful guy. One weekend his wife found him hanging in the attic.

My mother explained to my brother and me that his method revealed something of his motivation. Hanging yourself, she said, is an act of aggressive hostility, quite different from other forms of suicide. You are not just escaping from your own life—you are creating a ghastly tableau carefully calculated to shock and destroy the person who discovers you. That made sense to me, though I couldn't imagine why such a nice man would want to shock and destroy his wife. But isn't this how children learn the hard facts? Death of a salesman, indeed. George Sondergard dangling in his attic, eyes and tongue black and protruding, became part of the town's gothic lore, of which there was already an abundance.

For a while after my mother and Tim Durant were married, and before he bought the tall gray house, we rented a house owned by a family prominent in town, the Clevengers. The house was a replacement for another house that had sat on the same foundation but had burned to the ground. The old house had been three stories, ancient wood, and it went up like a Molotov cocktail. There had been only one person in the house on the night it burned, old Harold Clevenger, or "Grandpa." In the morning, when they searched the rubble, they found his body in the basement—headless. And they never found the head. This is absolutely true. I know it sounds like a rural urban legend, but it's not. It became one of my mother's favorites, and part of our own family lore when we lived in that house. Whenever my brother or I went down the basement stairs, my mother would call after us cheerfully: "Watch out for Grandpa Clevenger's head!"

In the summer of 1955, during one of my mother's many absences in the early years of her marriage to Durant, when my brother and I were farmed out and we both missed her acutely, it rained. And rained. And rained some more. Rain in the summer in Connecticut is as normal as sandstorms in the Kalahari, but this was just a little too much rain. The ground was saturated. Brooks and rivers ran high and muddy. Dams bulged.

Our town has high ground and low ground. You travel up a steep,

winding road to get to the "better" part of town. At the bottom of the
hill, you'll find stores and houses and a river. Not a mighty river, by any
means. Not even a river by some standards. A big wide brook, maybe a
foot deep at the most. That summer the brook became a furious wild
river when the narrow culverts under another bridge ten miles upstream
filled with debris, and water backed up behind it, turning the bridge into
a dam, which it was not built to be, and it exploded. The wall of raging
brown water swept down into our town and devastated it.

My brother and I were staying with friends of my mother's in a
neighboring township. We were never in danger. But we were taken to
see the aftermath of the flood. Angry rapids rushed over the pavement
atop the bridge at the bottom of the hill. Stores and houses stood in
brown water up to their second-floor windows. A dozen houses were
entirely gone. Amazingly, there were only two deaths: Mr. and Mrs.
Benoit (they pronounced it Ben-OYT) and their house had been swept
away. The bodies were found downriver, draped in the treetops.

Everyone knew that Mr. and Mrs. Benoit, though they lived under
one roof, had not exchanged a word in twenty years. Naturally, everyone wondered: When their house was being carried away by the flood-
waters, did they finally speak? Or did they adhere to their vow of
silence, and did it cost them their lives? Later, this became a game of
conjecture for my mother and brother and me when we rode in the car.
If Mr. and Mrs. Benoit spoke to each other that night, what did they
say? We'd invent conversations:

"Mildred, there's something I need to tell you."

"Fred, your pajamas are wet."

The town of my mother's lost memories is beautiful. It's in rolling
country in the foothills of the Berkshires. Parts of it look like a dreamscape New England, like stepping into a Christmas card, into someone's
nostalgic vision. There are hills, rivers, barns, stone walls, fields of hay and
flowers in the summer, frozen silent snowy woods in the winter. This
was the kingdom of her heart. She saw it for what was almost certainly
the last time when she left to come live in California. It's been almost
two years since Tom and I were there. And it's entirely possible that neither of us will ever go back again.

There's another cemetery in that town, a really old one. It's way off by itself along an empty road in the woods. It has graves dating back to the 1600s. Like all old cemeteries, there are a lot of very small tombstones with resting lambs carved on them and dates like: *March 27, 1746–April 15, 1747.* The last time I was there I went up and down the rows doing the simple arithmetic in my head. Sometimes it was done for me: *Wife and mother, Died 1763, aged 32 years, four months, three days.* Some of them made me look twice: *B. 1632, D. 1729.* I imagined the lives. And of course, I found more than one leaning, mossy time-weathered stone rasping at me waggishly in barely legible script, like a rogue lover throwing the bedclothes back, inviting me to come home, lie down under the green grass and close my eyes: *Hear ye friends, as you pass by; as you are now, so once was I . . .*

CHAPTER NINE

Judas Rising

October: We're riding in the Toyota, because the Volvo is undrivable, the front end rattling like roller skates in a washing machine. My mother snaps her basket open and rummages around. I know the basic contents of that basket, though it shifts a little from day to day: Her empty wallet with the picture of herself and Mike in it, her checkbook (which we gave back to her since we moved out of range of the liquor store), chewing gum, breath mints, cigarettes, matches, bandanna, nail scissors, and most poignant of all, her car and mailbox keys from Connecticut.

She brings out an old envelope or maybe a paper napkin or a corner of a newspaper with her handwriting all over it.

"I just have a short list of what I need," she says.

"I think we have everything you need, Mom." Eyes on the road, hands on the wheel, voice calm, I say to myself, mantra-like.

"Cigarettes."

"Bought you a carton day before yesterday."

"Cat food."

"I have tons of cat food. That's like asking the Pope if he has communion wafers."

"Vodka."

"Um, we're not drinking hard liquor these days. I have white wine for you."

"You have white wine?"

"Plenty."

"You're sure."

"I'm sure."

"Because I like a drink before dinner."

"Plenty of white wine, Mom. You've gotta stop worrying."

"But no vodka."

"Nope. No vodka." (Lie. There's actually a little cup of it on the backseat floor. I take a swig when she's looking out the window or searching in her basket. It's so easy.)

"What about cat food?"

"Plenty of cat food."

"And cigarettes?"

"Got a whole carton."

"What was the name of the doctor I went to last time I was out here?"

We're going to the supermarket in the next town. I dread these trips. Not because she makes scenes or wanders or anything like that. It's her desolation and impatience, telegraphing itself into my system. If I take her into the store, she walks around with me for a while and then quickly loses interest in the shopping and wants to go sit down and wait for me to finish. I wheel the cart around in a big hurry, making frequent passes toward the front of the store to check up on her, waiting for me on the bench. I know that her sense of time is all distorted. If I'm gone for five minutes it feels to her like an hour. With each pass of my cart, she waves urgently if she sees me, as if I've forgotten about her, abandoned her. If she doesn't see me, then I see her, a lonely lost sad woman watching the crowd, not sure where she is or why.

If I leave her in the car, she can doze, read, or do a crossword puzzle. But if I'm gone for more than a few minutes she'll get impatient and come looking for me, going from store to store in the shopping center. If she doesn't find me, then she'll forget which car she was in and get agitated. I can't leave her home alone, and if Mitch is there, I want to get her away from him so that he can have a few hours of peace and solitude.

Today, I've left her in the car with a magazine. I race around the store and get my shopping done. I'm in line. I reach into my purse for my wallet. It's not there. It must have fallen out in the car. I put my basket of groceries to one side and go out to the car. My mother's there, snoozing. I tell her I've left my wallet in the car somewhere. I look on the floor and under the seats. Nothing. I look in the glove compartment. I look under the seats again. My mother gets out of the car and starts to look with me. I get down on the pavement and look under the car. Nothing. I must have taken it out in the store somewhere and left it on a shelf. The wallet's full of credit cards, including my mother's. Rage starts to rise, at myself, for being such an unconscious feeble-minded self-sabotaging dolt.

I go into the store. I ask at the lost-and-found. The guy checks, shrugs apologetically. I make a circuit of the store, looking in all the places I stopped—the fruit bin, the vitamin shelf, the cat food department. Nothing. I go back out to the parking lot. My mother's still looking around under the seat and in the glove compartment. I ransack the car again. Nothing. I go to the cigarette store my mother and I were in before I went into the supermarket because I remember taking my wallet out there to show the woman my ID when I wrote a check. Nope, sorry. Nothing.

I go back into the supermarket, ask at the lost-and-found again, in vain, roam around the aisles some more, wild-eyed, a crazy person on the verge. I go back out to the car. I'm starting to froth at the mouth. I curse and curse and curse. I tear maps and papers from the glove compartment and hurl them around inside the car. I pound the steering wheel. I scream. People are looking.

My mother is trying to help. She's trying to make suggestions. She's trying to calm me. She's trying to be reasonable. But I'm scaring her. And even while I'm screaming and cursing and calling myself obscene names, some part of my consciousness calmly regards the disgraceful scene, and says: Bravo. Excellent performance. Keep up the good work. Rage and shout like a maniac, completely out of proportion to the event, scare the hell out of your poor mother, who knows perfectly well, despite her Alzheimer's, that she's become a plague and a burden on your life. Give her a good shocking dose of your frustration and resentment like a rock crashing through a window, like a blast from Hell.

When we get home, Mitch says the police called. My wallet was found about a mile from the shopping center, all cards present and accounted for. I call every card company and cancel anyway, because I've heard that sometimes a thief will copy down the numbers and then put the cards back in the wallet and leave it where it will be found. You think everything's fine, so you don't cancel your cards, and next thing you know you've bought someone a trip to Mexico or a fur coat. They'd barely be able to buy a T-shirt and a cup of coffee with my cards, which groaned with debt, but my mother's card would have been a gusher.

My voice is hoarse from screaming. I have to pretend to be my mother when I call her card company. I am assisted in my deception by my scratchy voice, which helps me believe I am someone else. Someone old. Someone very messed up and forgetful, who might be careless and dotty enough to blank out and lose a wallet in a parking lot. That part doesn't require much acting.

I was becoming something hideous, and I was the nucleus of her universe. If I went down the hall and shut the door to get dressed, she'd forget where I was, get anxious, come looking for me, call my name through the door. If I went and locked myself into the bathroom, she'd go outside, circle around, and tap-tap-tap on the window. Her need for me and her vigilance wore me down, down. I could scarcely work, hardly read a magazine article all the way through, let alone a book, and my exercise routine was in shambles. Mitch's demeanor grew daily more grim and green around the gills, and I could scarcely blame him. Most men would have walked long ago. We drank, had desperate sex, lost sleep. I ran myself ragged from the time I woke up until I closed my eyes trying to keep my mother away from him at the same time that I struggled to protect her from the knowledge that she had become—God have mercy on my soul for even forming the thought—old and in the way. I popped Valium day and night. Beautiful pharmaceutical; it unplugged my terror for a while so that I could function just a little. I think I might have keeled over dead without it, and that's the truth. Sometimes you have to Just Say Yes.

I started making secret phone calls. To Connecticut. To old-folks' homes. A vision was creeping into my head: I'd send her back. There were three places in or near her town. One of them was called Rose Haven, and it sounded as if it sprang full-blown from my own brow. A big old house in picturesque, historic Litchfield, a twenty-minute ride from the home town. I pictured her friends coming over, taking her out, to movies, to dinner, to openings at the art gallery. She'd be home. We would undo this ghastly mistake. The pleasant woman I spoke to said they had a room available. It cost about $120 a day, but I knew vaguely that my mother had some sort of long-term care policy that she'd taken out years before. And another place was only $75 a day, and much, much closer to her home!

I told Mitch and my brother. They were unanimous in their dissent: Her friends would be attentive at first, but they'd drift away. Not these people, I said. These are salt-of-the-earth Yankees. They don't drift away. What if there's an emergency? asked Mitch and Tom. There'd be long-distance phone calls in the middle of the night, desperate plane flights. It's a great fantasy, but it's not going to work.

I spoke to a couple of her friends and one of her doctors from home. The doctor was a really nice guy who was very fond of my mother. He listened with sympathy, then reminded me in the kindest way that people have their own lives. And one of her friends, a wonderful man who'd been particularly faithful and attentive for years and years after Mike's death, gave my idea some serious consideration. He didn't just dismiss it. But while we were talking about whether or not my mother's friends could or would pay lots of attention to her if I shipped her back there to a "home," he said something that sealed it for me. His words were real and true: People are fragile, he said. They can have the best of intentions, but they're fragile.

This, of course, was a fact I knew only too well by now.

So I started to look around my own neighborhood.

There's a new and pleasant assisted-living place not so far away. It's called the Hostel. I know it well because an older friend of mine had a stroke and spent some time there. It's in a woodsy setting, is architect-designed and landscaped. The food is excellent. There are birds and blooming rhododendrons. Every room has a private deck. I call. The price is not astronomical. We'd discovered by now that her long-term care policy would not cover assisted living, only a full-on nursing home, two little words that fill me with the same kind of dread as would, say, "brain tumor" or "Algerian jail." We know she isn't ready for that yet.

My brother, by now seriously worried about me and Mitch, says we'll find the money to pay for an assisted-living place even if it means the family assets won't last long. There's only one little problem, though. The Hostel is full, and the waiting list is five to six months long.

Five to six months? Impossible, I think. I'll be dead meat by then.

So we look at what else is available. There's a nursing home and two other small assisted-living places in the town up the road. None of them is a hellhole. Far from it. True hellholes are usually an urban phenomenon. In cities, there can occur a kind of malignant anonymity. Places are too big, there's way too much turnover in the mostly underpaid staff. Untrained minimum-wage workers, bitter about their own raw-deal lives, are often free to take out their frustrations on helpless senile people. You can get away with things in the city that you can't in a small town, where family and friends visit more often, where news travels fast. And the appearance of a place is not always a reliable indicator—Mitch once worked inspecting nursing homes and similar facilities for the state of California, and he said some of the worst places he saw, where people were starved and abused and lying in shit and bedsores, had the fanciest facades. Fancy facades are what the places up here in our rural venue definitely do not have, with the exception of the Hostel.

One of the places in particular is run by really good kind people. That's the sort of thing you know in a small town. The food is excellent and there's plenty of it. It's clean. The old folks are cared for with compassion and patience. But we go and look at it, and I see instantly that it's out of the question. Why? Because it's so goddamned tragically dumpy and pathetic-looking. My mother's taste and artistic eye had been superb. There were no plaid sofas, crocheted afghans, ruffled lampshades, doilies or overhead light fixtures blighting the aesthetic landscape of my childhood. And it wasn't because she was rich. Money was always a little tight after Tim Durant left the scene. She just knew what was good.

And so it is that I recoil from the humble little board-and-care

homes in our neighboring town. I reject one of them without even getting out of the car. I can see everything I need to see through the wind-
shield: A jerry-built collection of wooden buildings and trailers, it sits
about ten feet from a busy road where huge diesel logging trucks roar
by at sixty miles an hour. The old folks sit at a big picture window facing the road, right there in full view in their Barca-Loungers and wheelchairs like mannequins in a store window. Dismal with a capital "D."
Even if she were in a coma I couldn't put her there.

The other one will take her right away, but after we tour it one rainy
afternoon, after we see the sad, cramped sitting-room with the giant
color TV and the hideous couch and the low ceiling and the braided rugs
and the prints of little girls with watering cans and bonnets on the green
walls, and after we see the dingy little dining area with small ugly formi-
ca-topped tables, and especially after we see the room that she would
share with an old lady who, even though she's sound asleep, is obviously
someone sweet and nice whose peaceful life would be shattered—after
we see all this, I want to put my head in an oven, preferably gas.

It wasn't just the effect that the end-of-the-road shabbiness had on
me. It was the effect that I knew it would have on her. Ugly surroundings and bad taste aren't just an annoyance—they are oppressive, can
actually be conducive to mental illness, particularly for someone like my
mother. Damaged and demented though she was, her aesthetic eye was
intact. You'd think that dementia would make all of that irrelevant, but
in a way, it intensifies it. Dementia tends to remove filters and inner gov-
ernors—like forbearance and equanimity, for instance. She would have
been abandoned and angry anyway and the plaid sofa and green walls
and low ceilings would have assaulted her like a bad drug trip. She'd flip
out in the first five minutes. I knew, I just knew, that the staff could no
more handle her than they could handle a bucking bronco in their parlor. We got her on the waiting list for the Hostel and hunkered down
for the wait.

Her insurance company said that they could upgrade her long-term
care policy to include assisted living—if she qualified. To determine if
she qualified, a certified nurse would come to the house for an evaluation. The nurse would be checking her physical health and her cogni-

tive capacity. A physically healthy person with not-too-far-advanced dementia, like my mother, is the ideal candidate for assisted living. But like any medical insurance policy, you have to prove that you don't need it before you can get it. Any whiff of a pre-existing condition—like cognitive impairment—and you can kiss it goodbye.

They'd also be checking her medical records. Technically, there had never been any diagnosis of Alzheimer's, because, of course, there had been no postmortem. Nor had we drilled a hole in her head to take samples. What we had was the expert opinion of the psychologist, not quite the same thing as a diagnosis. In any case, we'd been using the word freely for months and months, and her records were littered with it, even when a particular doctor visit had nothing to do with her mental state. If she'd gone to a doctor about her stomach, or her feet, or her ear, there was that word: Alzheimer's.

We made a mighty effort to expunge the word from her records. We called the various doctors. We said that the word actually had come from us, and we were certainly not qualified to make a diagnosis, and so there was no reason for it to be an official part of her records. They had to agree that that was so. It got removed here and there, but by now it would have been like taking the sugar out of a cake.

Meanwhile, the nurse sent by the insurance company was coming. They told us that for the cognition evaluation, my mother and the nurse would have to be alone together, presumably so we wouldn't be giving her cues or hints. Fuck that, we said. No way were we going to be shut out of witnessing a test that might be deciding whether we lived or died.

We coached my mother first.

"What year is it?"

"1989."

"No. It's 1999. When were you born?"

"1922."

"Right. How old are you now?"

"Eighty."

"No, Mom. Seventy-seven."

"Seventy-seven."

"What month is this?"

"June."

"No. October. Say it out loud: October."

"October."

"Who's the president?"

"Clinton."

"Right! Excellent!"

And so on. We'd ask her the same questions again a few hours later. She actually seemed to retain a few things. We figured we had about a fifty-fifty chance. And we had a plan for listening in on the interview.

The nurse arrived at the appointed time. She was one of these frighteningly businesslike people who seem to me like a different species. She was young and pretty and obviously pregnant, but she was as steely as a Marine Corps Major. She knew how to make polite small talk, but she also had perfect immunity to any kind of chit-chat designed to elicit her sympathy and influence her report. She came into the house, met my mother, made a few pleasantries, the minimum required by civility, and then asked questions about my mother's health. Soon it was time for the cognition test. I got up, said I thought the cottage would be the best place for them to go and that I wanted to step out there for a minute to make sure everything was in order.

We have two phone lines with cordless extensions. I had taken both of them, a black one and a white one, out to the cottage before the nurse arrived. I had also unplugged the corded extension to one of them inside the house, silencing it. When I excused myself from the table, Mitch detained the nurse for a few minutes. I went out to the cottage, called the white phone from the black phone, clicked the white phone to "talk" and hid it on top of a cabinet. Keeping the line open, I put the black phone in my pocket and went back to the house. The nurse and my mother went out to the cottage.

Mitch and I took the black phone upstairs, where we had a good aerial view of the front door of the cottage. We huddled together and listened. Our bugging device was working perfectly. We could hear the scrape of feet, voices, words, clear and distinct.

My poor mother. This nurse was the kind of person she once would have deconstructed without mercy on the written page. Now the woman was deconstructing my mother. We groaned and made faces while we listened:

"Who's the president?"

"Carter." (At least she didn't say Roosevelt.)

"What year is it?"

"1997."

She did amazingly well on some things. Count backward from one hundred by sevens, the woman said. Mitch and I silently cheered my mother on while we listened. Yeah! Go, Mom!

"One hundred. Ninety-three. Eighty-six. Seventy-nine . . ."

With some parts of the test, we had no clue:

"Please draw a clock face that says ten of eleven." And: "I'm going to show you a design. I want you to look at it. Then I'm going to cover it up and I want you to draw it from memory."

She flunked. We had to wait a week or so for the results, because Nursie sure as hell didn't give us any kind of clue when they emerged from the cottage, but she flunked.

So we took a hard look at her old policy. We found something it would pay for that we thought might help us: Certified Nurse Assistants to come to the house and provide "companionship." We decided to try it. The idea was to keep her occupied and entertained, we fervently hoped, and away from us for a few hours of respite. Allen had another job and wasn't available. There was a local adult activities program for dementia patients that was affordable, but I rejected it. I'd stuck my nose in a couple of times and thought it was totally lame. Singalongs, jigsaw puzzles, idiotic arts and crafts. There were mentally retarded people in the mix, too. Even at this late date, I was still trying to live up to my mother's legacy. And I was deep in that big Egyptian river: *My* world-class mother on the same level with those people? One thing for sure—damaged though she was, I knew she wouldn't put up with it for more than an hour.

The other reason we'd rejected it, probably the more compelling reason, was because although they'd send a bus around to pick her up right at the door, she'd have to be dressed, fed and ready to go at 8:30 in the morning. I would have had to be up by at least 7:00 to get her ready. I was getting to sleep (passing out, more precisely) around 2:00 or 3:00 A.M. these days. The night hours after we put my mother to bed were the only private time Mitch and I had. Those precious extra hours of sleep in the morning, even one or two, were the only thing standing between me and a complete psychotic breakdown.

November: The first CNA they send is about eighteen, but a tough little cookie. My mother is polite when we introduce the girl to her. "Oh, she's really nice," the girl says about my mother. I leave them alone together in the cottage. I go into the house and sit down at my computer. Twenty or thirty minutes go by, when I'm levitated from my chair by a screech of rage which, though I hadn't heard it for years, is what my subconscious was waiting for: "Leave me ALONE!"

So we try having the girl take my mother away. Take her anywhere, we say—for rides, to the beach, the movies. She likes to get out. She likes action. Just get her out of here for a while. She's always complaining that she's stuck here and never goes anywhere. So off they go, my mother with a shopping list, this time one I myself have contrived, and a few dollars in her pocket. "Don't let her buy booze," we warn the girl.

An hour later the phone rings. My mother, demanding that we come pick her up, that she's been abducted, that she has no idea where she is. I reassure her, tell her all is well, that we know where she is. Maybe an hour or two later, the exhausted girl brings her back. After she's gone, my mother tells a wild tale about being dumped in the middle of nowhere and having to hitchhike back to the house.

We give up the experiment after a couple of weeks. It's much less harrowing to just keep her at home. She's back on the window seat, or shuffling back and forth between the house and the cottage, all day, every day, weeping, little flurries of sobs erupting out of nowhere, asking about stomach medicines and doctors, complaining that she's stuck here and never goes anywhere.

The rain comes, as it does in November on the northern California coast, and the dark winter months stretch in front of us like a miniature eternity. Way off in the distance, like a tantalizing shining mirage of paradise, is the bright beautiful day when the Hostel will call and tell us the wait is over.

It's a day I yearn for, and just about equally, fear and dread. Because I will have to betray my mother.

People ask me sometimes why my brother didn't take care of my mother. They also expect, as a matter of course, resentment on my part, bitterness. I've heard a lot about sibling enmity. I know it's as common as mud and a big complication in a lot of people's adult lives. I listen to friends savaging their brothers and sisters the way they would a bad ex-spouse. They seem to have their hooks in each other's lives in a destructive, chronic sort of way.

Tom and I fought when we were kids. A lot. It drove my mother crazy. Right around when she split from Durant, when money was scarce and she was frustrated in love, a single parent with no one to share the load, we were at our squabbling, whining, selfish pre-teen worst. We started up any time, any place, in the car, in public, at home. She tried sitting us down once when I was ten and he was twelve and having a calm, rational discussion about our endless fighting and its effect on her, but the session deteriorated into the two of us bickering and ended with her running from the room and up the stairs. *Boom-boom-boom-boom-boom!*

Somewhere in that era, maybe a year or so later, we started up our five thousand two hundred forty-seventh fight. My mother burst into the room in her nightgown, a flyswatter in her hand and tears streaming down her face. "*Stop it, stop it, stop it!*" she sobbed, flailing at us with the flyswatter, which of course didn't hurt us at all, but we did stop. She'd made an impression. Sometimes this is what it takes to penetrate the self-absorption of children—a demonstration of grownup pain. That reminder again: Huh? Wuh? *She* has feelings?

We quit fighting fairly abruptly when we were teenagers, and haven't fought since. We've been damned nice to each other over the years, sympathetic, always on the other's side. Friends. Pretty unusual, I guess.

I don't resent Tom not taking on my mother, because I didn't want him to. The Durant years were a lot harder on him than they were on me. Durant robbed him. The bastardly psychological abuse of a super-smart, deep, thoughtful boy were costly to my brother in insidious ways that he's still figuring out. The Durant harangues and early-life letdowns by my mother rearranged my brother's wiring, as he himself put it, so that relations between them are as complex as the labyrinth where Theseus killed the Minotaur. By comparison, my love for my mother is simpler, more streamlined. Vastly fewer detours and roadblocks. I know it would have been twice as painful for my brother to try to care for her as it was for me, and I'm glad to have been able to spare him that. People stare at me incredulously when I tell them all this, but it's the truth.

After Mike's death, my mother attached to my brother in a longing sort of way that was intensely sad for him and fraught with conflict— an awkward desire to have him "replace" Mike as the masculine figure in her life, a tragic reversal of her one-time disdain for grown sons who lived with their mothers. The terrible pull of her desolation and yearning was a living, breathing thing. Any time he wanted to, he could have just said, "Okay, Mom, I'm coming home," and she would have rejoiced. And there he'd be: driving her around, looking at his *Playboy*s, getting a big belly. Getting old.

He does his part. He's the one who had the spine to step in and rescue her from herself before it was too late, and he's the one who guards the modest family account, maintains an honorable ethical balance between seeing to it that my mother is cared for and—barring the unforeseen—trying to give us a financial future. I'm happy to leave the responsibility to him, *glad* to leave it to him, and I trust him totally. If I'd been the one in charge of the business end of things, my mother would probably have burned her house down by now, been committed to an asylum in Waterbury, or Torrington, or Bridgeport, and every penny would be gone.

Or else, more likely, *I'd* be back there in her house with her, hiding the car keys, hiding the liquor, a bottle of my own hidden in a wastebasket, chasing after her, listening at night for her footsteps, listening to church bells and katydids and my heart inside my chest ticking my life away. Trying to remember Mitch's face. California dreaming. *Shiny black perforated tie-up shoes on my feet peeking over the edge of a freshly dug grave . . .*

January: It's evening, about 10:15. My mother and I watch a show about a guy on death row who's been trying for fifteen years to prove his innocence. While we're watching, I keep an eye on the clock. Can't let this go on too long, I think. Have to get her out of here at a reasonable hour. But this is a fascinating show, and my mother's engaged, a fairly rare occurrence nowadays. And we're having what they call "quality time," an even rarer occurrence.

Mitch is upstairs reading. He's tired. So am I. We did a lot of hard work that day—painting, cleaning, hauling junk. We worked as a team, almost enjoyed the work, made real progress. He's occupied, enjoying the peace and solitude, I'm sure. I usually have my mother out of here and in bed by 9:30 or so, but tonight we got involved in this show. It's going on longer than I thought it would. I start to feel a little anxiety around the edges. Will Mitch be annoyed? And I think: You're being most ungenerous to believe he might be so unreasonable. He'll cut you some slack after a hard but productive day like this one, the same way you would for him. He seems to be in a good mood—earlier, he'd made a little joke about falling on the floor from exhaustion, and we'd all laughed.

The show ends at 10:30. Mitch is still upstairs. I hustle my mother out of there and into her cottage. I run a bath, lay out her breakfast things, wash some dirty dishes, get her into her nightgown, kiss her good-night, pull the curtains. I'm back in the house by 10:45.

Whew, I think. Pretty good. It's not even 11:00 yet. I'm in the kitchen. I hear Mitch come in. I turn around, ready to give him a friendly it-was-a-hard-day-but-we-got-a-lot-done-and-maybe-there's-a-light-at-the-end-of-the-tunnel-after-all greeting. Instead, my innards contract. He's angry.

"Why did you take so long to get your mother the hell out of here?"

I try to tell him about the show, that it was really interesting, that my mother was absorbed, that I wanted to relax for a while.

"Besides," I say, "it's not all that late. Look at the clock! It's not that late!"

He doesn't respond. Ominous silence. I go and look out the front window, heart pounding, trying to stay calm. Then I hear his voice behind me, quiet and matter-of-fact.

"Did you get any beer today?"

"No," I say. "I'm sorry. I forgot."

The words are barely out of my mouth when I hear a loud crash of something thrown and broken. I don't even turn around to see what it was. I bolt, out the door and down the driveway and out to the road. I think: I'm at the end. I have no one, no one in the world. My mother has lost her mind and my lover has gone mad, throws things and lets me run out into the night and doesn't come after me. My brother is a thousand miles away. I could go to friends' houses, but I don't want to. The idea of blubbering and whining and gut-spilling is repugnant. What the hell good would it do anyway?

There's no need to go to anyone's house. It's remote and rural here, zero crime, completely safe to roam around alone at any time of the day or night. An anachronism and a luxury, especially for me on that particular evening. Because that's exactly what I do. It's mild, the sky is full of stars and the moon is up. I go down the hill and into town. I'm going where I can sit for a while, alone, where no one will look at me or ask questions. I head for the cemetery.

I wander down the rows. I find by chance the grave of an old man I met once or twice, the father of someone I know. There's a photo on the tombstone, of the old man when he was young and a boxer. I look at the ghostly picture in the pale moonlight: He's bare-chested, in satin shorts, gloves up in the classic pugilist pose of yesteryear.

I sit on the grass, lean against the tombstone for the better part of an hour. Heaving spasmodic sobs rolling up out of the pit of despair gradually subside. I walk home.

My mother's cottage is dark and quiet. Inside the house, it's silent. I put my stealthy ear to the bedroom door: heavy snores. I don't dare go in. It might wake him up.

My mother's been on the waiting list at the Hostel for five weeks. Or is it six? I look at the calendar. No, just five weeks. It might be another fifteen. Or twenty. And I think: I should go over there and put a few discreet pillows over some faces. Move that list along.

Because it's them or me.

CHAPTER TEN

Thin Ice

February: It's not even dark yet, and I'm drunk. Today we left my mother at the Hostel. Our beat-up old ugly brown Toyota was completely covered with pink petals from the flowering plum tree it was parked under. The car looked as if it had participated in some sort of ceremony. Something Japanese having to do with spring. Something festive and whimsical.

I feel like Judas Iscariot. The call from the Hostel came day before yesterday, out of the blue, weeks earlier than we'd expected. Today had been a day of lies and subterfuge. Our battle plan had been in place ever since we got her on the waiting list: Mitch would take my mother out for three hours or so. Shopping, errands. The instant they left, I sprang into action.

I dragged a big suitcase out from under the bed. Went out to her cottage. Plundered her drawers and closets. Made instant selections: These pants, and these, and these, clean and presentable. These pants, and these, spotted, frayed, pathetic-looking. The good stuff into the suitcase, the sad stuff into a pile. Same with sweaters, shirts, underwear, shoes. The freight of sentiment at the sight of certain articles of clothing threatening to overwhelm me. A cuff on one of her sweaters, artfully rolled to conceal the hole. A shirt she loved and wore for years and years, now stained and grubby. All signs of her slippage and my failure. She was, and still is, a snappy dresser. Even depressed and demented, she puts together a jaunty outfit every morning. It just kills me.

But I surprise myself with my fortitude. I make my selections, click the suitcase shut, stuff the worn dirty things in a box. I'll wash some, throw some out.

Then it's a sweep through the bathroom. Here's where I waver and slug down a shot of vodka. There's a Japanese word, *kawaisoo*, which, roughly translated, means "the pity of things." Here are prime examples: her lipstick, tweezers, toothpaste, hairspray, little bottles of makeup, combs, hairbrushes. The bathroom has been a source of unhappiness for me all along. We never quite finished it when we did the conversion, so desperate were we to move her out of the house and into the cottage, pressed for money and time and starved for privacy. When we painted the floor we were in a big hurry and never got around to the corners and edges. We didn't put up trim, and there's a curtain instead of a door. Stray pieces of rug were nailed to the floor. The rug is now grungy, the unpainted corners of the floor dusty and fuzzy. I get out of there as fast as I can.

I grab the handsome African blanket from her bed. Her bed, which she always neatly makes, every morning, that she'd made that morning not knowing she probably would not be sleeping in it ever again. Her books and magazines and crossword puzzles. It's all her little efforts at maintaining that unhinge me.

But I do it. Grab her folding chaise, her small Oriental rug, a tape player with the Big Band tape in it, a TV table. Toss it all into the car. I go back into the cottage and pause in front of the photos she's put up on the wall: my brother and me as children and adults, old friends, and Mike, Mike, Mike. No pictures for now, I decide. Especially, no pictures of Mike. My overworked tear ducts give a fatigued tingle at the sight of them.

Mike, I ask one photo of him, the profile shot where he's outdoors wearing his tam o'shanter and looking very glamorous indeed, quite unintentionally, am I doing the right thing? I'm doing what a local psychiatrist advised my mother to do. Even though you're an atheist, the psychiatrist had said, and you have no belief that Mike is waiting for you in the hereafter or watching over you or any of that, you still have an image of him in your mind. And you can consult that image. You can ask it what Mike would say or do in a certain situation. And in that way you are communing with him. I remember thinking: Damn! That's a useful piece of advice. It was lost on my mother, forgotten as soon as it was said, but it wasn't lost on me. The image of Mike in my head, the wise compassionate person I remember, said, Yes, you're doing the right thing.

At least, I think that's what the image said.

She'd been in the cottage for only about eight months. How utterly fantastic to think that I once believed she might be there for eight years. The cozy haven we tried to make it turned gradually and sadly into a solitary confinement cell. That's how she saw it. Squalor and clutter took over. Nothing to call the Elder Abuse Hotline about, but not the level of dignity she deserved. Her housekeeping abilities slipped inch by inch, and so the job of keeping the place decent fell by increments to me, along with the cooking, and I was doing an inadequate job. I was also doing an inadequate job of keeping her hair, clothes and body clean. If I didn't lead her to the sink and wash her hair for her, it didn't get done. And I didn't do it often enough. What I had feared for a long time was beginning to happen: I was getting so burnt out I was neglecting her.

A senile person with dirty hair is a tragedy. It embarrassed me, aroused pity, sorrow and contempt in me, and I loathed those feelings and myself for feeling them. She has really nice hair, and when it's fresh and fluffy everything about her seems improved. So first I'd clean out her sink, full of stinky cat food cans, wet cigarette butts, crusty forks and greasy frying pans. Then I'd announce that it was time to wash her hair. But I just washed it yesterday, she'd say. Um—I don't think so, I'd say. C'mon. It's easy. Here's a towel. Let's do it. If I had short hair like yours I'd wash it every day.

And she'd bend over the sink while I sprayed her head. It made me sad to see the vulnerable nape of her neck. Then I'd fill my hand with shampoo and rub it into her hair. I knew she liked the touching and attention, but I found it disturbing to feel the contours of her skull. It brought unpleasantly vivid images to my morbidly imaginative mind.

I'd think of her damaged brain just a centimeter or so from my fingers. And I hated myself for feeling that reluctance to touch her head. Touching, of course, was one of the things she ached for most since Mike's death.

And when I made her take a bath, the sight of her naked body was tragic and disturbing to me, too. Though her muscles were atrophied, I could still see, in the line of her legs and the curve of her waist, the remnants of her beauty. The body Mike had loved. One night, months and months before we'd moved out of the old house and she was still living in her apartment a block away, she'd been undressing, and was standing there in her sweater and underpants, and I'd seen the gentle curve of her belly, and when I got home that night after putting her to bed I lay on the floor and wept helplessly for an hour. No one loves her anymore, I thought. No one in the whole world. Only me. And Tommy. We're it.

The big picture is dreadful, but in the end it's the little stuff that makes you cry Uncle. The Chinese perfected the art of bloodless torture centuries ago. It was so much cleaner, more civilized, and oh, so exquisitely painful: water dripping on your forehead until you went mad. Tedium and repetition are what finally make you crack, void all your grand plans and noble intentions. The senile person's world is a shrunken, fretful place, but it's all the person has, and so the vexingly trivial things in it are worried and worried and worried like an old dog chew, and if the person is someone you really love, like your mother, for instance, then you're sucked right in there with her.

And when I say little stuff, I mean little stuff. There was a routine we went through almost every day: She'd pick up, say, a rubber band or maybe a paperclip from the floor and ask: "Where does this go?" As soon as I'd shown her what to do with the rubber band or the paperclip, she'd find a plastic fork or a paper bag. "Where does this go?" Then a broken comb, or a piece of string, a bottle cap, a cork, an empty can, a pencil, until I wanted to shriek. And the capriciousness of her visual perception was altogether baffling: She could see these tiny, insignificant bits of trash, but her basket could be sitting right in front of her, invisible.

It's a conundrum. So much of the demented person's behavior is irritating, but the relentless repetition and obsession with minutiae become infuriating. Since the dementia is beyond the control of the afflicted person, it's never appropriate to react irritably, but unless you are Mother Teresa, you react irritably. Sometimes you blow your top. And the more burdensome and maddening the suffering person's demands, the more you try to escape, and the more persistent and urgent the demands become. And so the heartbreak multiplies and mutates, until you don't recognize yourself anymore.

She can't help it, you tell yourself. She can't help it. But neither can you. I remember one really awful day, my mother out in the driveway in the rain, her hair in her face like a madwoman's. She'd been pestering Mitch with some question or other, over and over, while he tried to fix a broken car, and he'd finally bellowed at her to leave him alone.

"You don't want me!" she shouted. "You don't want me!" The very words she spoke to Tim Durant more than forty years before.

I watched through the window. Before dementia, she and Mitch had been good pals. She adored him. He was gallant with her.

And here's what it's come to.

In the old days, when I was in trouble or needed help, I'd pick up the phone and call my mother. Every once in a while in the middle of all this I still get the crazy impulse: the Connecticut area code, the familiar little tune her number played on the touch-tone, her voice.

Of course, I can't. I grieve for her exactly as if she'd died. She's gone, I've lost her, but I'm still responsible for her living, breathing body and the ghosts in her head.

Sometimes I feel like one of those ghosts. I think back on a morning about a month before: I wake to the sound of my mother's voice in the hall outside the bedroom. I jump up and open the door. There she is, dressed and groomed, talking on the phone, leaving a message on an answering machine. My answering machine. She's using one of my phones to call the other one right there in the same house. It's a chilling little moment, not unlike the moment in the movie *The Eye of the Needle* when the heroine discovers that her lover, played by Donald Sutherland, is a Nazi spy. She walks in on him while he's in the middle of sending a radio message in German. He goes on with his transmission, calmly, coolly, terrifyingly, looking right at her. My mother looks right at me while she finishes her message, her voice perfectly normal: Anyway, dear, I'd like to see you. Come and pick me up as soon as you can.

Had I become a ghost? Had she? Or had we become ghosts together?

I finish loading the car with her things. One last detail: I go into the house, lug our spare TV out to the cottage, set it up on the table next to her magazines and typewriter and put the bouquet of flowers that had been on her own TV on top of it. It's a ruse, designed to trick the eye. So that when Mitch brings her home, she won't notice anything different.

Our wait had turned out to be less than three months. I'd been taking her over to the Hostel regularly, for "activities"; singing, memory games, an occasional lunch. The place will be familiar to her, I thought. I desperately fervently hoped.

No, I'm not good at betrayal. You don't want me as your general, as the one to inspire the troops when hard action must be taken. I'd fretted obsessively over how, when the moment came, we'd actually take her there, leave her there. And I'd fretted over how to make it work. She'd drive them crazy with her stomach. It won't work, it won't work, it won't work, said the reliable old voice of doom and dread.

Of course it'll work, of course it'll work, of course it'll work, said the voice of desperate hope. They know what they're doing. This is their business. There may be a little "adjustment" period, naturally, but then she'll like it! She'll get away from me and Mitch, two sorry, evil-tempered permanently hungover hollowed-out husks of human beings if ever there were any.

I drive to the Hostel and set up her room. Clothes in the drawers and closet. TV on the table, Oriental rug on the floor, toiletries in the bathroom. Fresh flowers. We'll take her there for dinner that night, walk her down the hall to her room, and then . . .

When my mother and Mike were getting ready to go on their first Audubon expedition in the mid-seventies, and word got out that they were going to go by car and camp out, a cranky old guy in their town rolled his eyes and remarked, "Well, there goes that marriage." No doubt he was picturing himself and *his* wife on a months-long camping and car trip, which would have been disastrous indeed.

My mother and Mike had the time of their lives. Being together in a car and a tent for months on end was bliss for them. That's the kind of marriage they had—they really, really preferred each other's company to anyone else's. It's rare, but it happens. They never got bored or fed up with each other. I remember being at a big noisy New Year's party in Connecticut sometime in the 1980s. My mother and I went together, and Mike was going to meet us there later. He'd been gone since morning on some business or other. When he arrived, my mother was talking with people and I was about ten feet away, up on a couple of steps, so I had a panoramic view of the party. I watched Mike come in the back door and head through the packed kitchen. He was looking for her. She saw him and he saw her at the same time, across the proverbial crowded room. They smiled with spontaneous joy and headed straight for one another, hugged and kissed. These were people who'd been together maybe sixteen years by then, and who'd been apart that day for a few hours. I saw.

They traveled a total of thirteen months on the Audubon trip, with occasional pit stops at home in between. Then they spent another solid year and a half or so collaborating on the manuscript. This was just before the dawn of the Age of the Word Processor, so their two typewriters—Mike's electric and my mother's manual—pounded away in counterpoint between the top and bottom floors of the house. They conferred, argued, agreed, wrote, rewrote, cut, replaced, revised, argued, conferred, worked and worked and worked.

The book came out in 1980. It was a masterpiece, got rave reviews, won some prizes, but like a lot of masterpieces, it pretty much sank beneath the waves. It was a combination a little too familiar to most writers—lack of publicity, a failing publishing house, poor management.

My mother was bitter. Not catastrophically, acutely bitter. It was a gradual, cumulative disappointment. There was, for instance, talk of a public television production based on their book. The bicentennial of Audubon's birth, 1985, was coming up. There was a veritable Audubon revival going on. The timing was perfect. My mother and Mike would be consultants, might even appear as themselves in reenactments of some of their adventures. The book would come out in a new edition. It would have a second life.

Like too many great ideas, this one fizzled and flopped. My mother's disappointment was not that the book would fail to make her rich and famous. It was that she was proud of their superb work and she wanted the recognition. I suppose there are some writers out there who are satisfied to write in a vacuum, but they're scarce as trumpeter swans. My mother was not one of them. She had a rare gift, and she knew it.

The final entry in the 617-page book is hers. By this time she and Mike had traveled from Labrador to the Dry Tortugas, from Pennsylvania to Texas in Audubon's footsteps. He had long since ceased to be an abstract concept, a colorful but very dead historical figure. As they tracked him all over the country for more than a year, dug up obscure information and local stories and delved into his letters and journals, this complicated Frenchman from another century came almost eerily to life. They found themselves deeply entangled emotionally with Audubon and his family, especially his benighted wife, Lucy.

Audubon's travels ended in New York City in the 1840s. He died and was buried there in 1851. The family had a home at 155th Street and Riverside Drive. It's hard to imagine the rural Eden that address was in those days—forty acres of shade trees, orchards, vegetable gardens, a stable, poultry yards, a brook with a waterfall, fishing in the river. It was a little bit different in 1979 when my mother and Mike went there.

It was a melancholy pilgrimage for them. This was Audubon's last stop, and so it was theirs too. They went to his grave, in the cemetery of a Gothic church a few blocks from where his house had been. My mother had a tough time holding back the tears. Her reaction took her by surprise. She wrote:

> . . . at that moment I realize for the first time that I know more about John James Audubon than I do about anyone else in the world, except myself. I know more about him than I do about my husband, my children, my parents. I've read his journals, his mail, his anecdotes, his essays, the complete accounting—the vanities, lies and blather, follies and furors, the triumphs and the failures. We've stood in his tracks, tramped

*his woods and marshes, his riverbanks and seashores, climbed
his hills, seen his vistas, slept under his skies and his moon.
We have followed him down the arches of the years, and this
moment, at his gravesite, is the day of his death. It's done.*

She hid her welling tears behind her dark glasses, and wandered away
to explore other parts of the cemetery, away, as she put it:

> *. . . from the image of self weeping at Audubon's tomb. (There
> would have been a tableau for the yardmen and anyone look-
> ing out the windows of the parish office.)*

Audubon was sixty-five when he died. A few years before, he had
been at work on his final oeuvre, *Quadrupeds of America,* but was unable
to finish the project. The problem? Alzheimer's. My mother was afraid
that she'd burst into tears at Audubon's grave. When I read what she
wrote about Audubon's decline, I'm in danger of a fit of intemperate
blubbering myself, but not for John James Audubon . . .

She describes how Audubon's old friend, patron and fellow adven-
turer John Bachman tried to penetrate the fog drifting over Audubon's
mind: "Wake up and work as you used to!" Bachman implored, begged,
raged. For naught. My mother wrote:

> *. . . the unthinkable was coming to pass. Audubon now spoke
> of himself as a "poor old man" . . . and then—as though the
> drives and passions that possessed him for a lifetime had
> burned out the circuits of his brain—JJA drifted off into the
> never-never land of senility . . .*

Bachman visited the household around 1848, and reported the sor-
rowful truth in a letter to his wife. He said:

> *His is indeed a most melancholy case. I have often sat down
> sad & gloomy in witnessing a ruin, that I had seen in other
> years in order & neatness, but the ruins of a mind once bright
> & full of imagination is still more melancholy to the observer
> . . . the outlines of his countenance & his general robust form
> are there, but the mind is all in ruins . . . imagine to yourself
> a crabbed restless uncontrollable child, worrying and bothering
> every one & you have not a tythe of a description of this poor
> old man . . .*

I couldn't have put it better myself.

Talking about her disappointment with *On the Road*'s performance years later, my mother pointed to the final couple of paragraphs of the book. There's a quote from a granddaughter of Audubon's when she was reminiscing about her childhood at the Audubon family home on the Hudson. The granddaughter talks about the joys of being a child roaming and roving free in this idyllic setting, swimming, fishing, climbing trees, until she heard the call on summer evenings that meant it was time to come inside, that the day was done: "Sunset, children!"

My mother and Mike went to the spot where the Audubon house had stood. It was demolished in 1932, after it had fallen into dereliction and decay, to make way for the Riverside Drive viaduct. She describes the superstructures of masonry, steel and concrete that occupy the place now, the blighted urban cityscape, and the two of them trying to see through all of that and visualize the land the way it once was. These are the final lines of the book:

> Upstream, the George Washington Bridge and the little red lighthouse on the promontory at its feet. Downstream, a pall of smoke. Something is burning on the Jersey Shore. A jogger huffs by. The day wanes. We head home.
>
> Sunset, children.

She knew what fine writing that was, knew it was sheer inspiration to end their amazing saga with those two words.

"God damn it," she said to me about five years after the book came out and when it was clear that it was more or less destined for obscurity. I remember her leaning over the table, speaking almost through clenched teeth with intensity: "God damn it. I wanted to finally show people *what I can do.*"

In 1987, Mike traveled to Ecuador and went up into the Andes. It was a nature expedition of some sort. I don't know why my mother wasn't along on that trip. No doubt she had pressing work to finish.

Something happened in the high altitude: Mike had a crisis, got acutely short of breath. He came close to collapsing. A few months later, back home in Connecticut, he had a bout of atrial fibrillation that took him and my mother to the emergency room in the middle of the night. He developed a chronic cough.

Various misdiagnoses followed. Pneumonia was one of them, and that great vague when-in-doubt catch-all, stress. It wasn't pneumonia, though, nor was it stress. If only. It took a young cardiologist friend to finally figure it out over a year later: blood clots in his pulmonary arteries. A lot of them, some of them years and years old, collecting insidiously. The source? His arm.

Thinking about Mike's arm leads me straight into a Sargasso Sea of philosophical conundrums. Whatever genetic combination occurred when sperm met egg and made Mike the man that he was also made the arm. His intelligence, compassion and lucidity were part of the same package that included the vascular defects that caught up with him and took him down way too soon. But in addition to being part of what was ineffably Mike, the arm, his fatal flaw, informed his thought, vision, character. He strengthened the arm, and the arm, even though it wound up killing him, strengthened him.

I sure wish Mike and my father had had a chance to know each other. They talked briefly on the phone a few times, but that was it. They could have liked each other. Plenty of dissimilarities, to be sure—my father would no more have sung "Lulu's Back in Town" in a loud jolly voice while accompanying himself on the guitar in a roomful of well-lubricated partygoers than he'd have gone out in public with his pants off, and I seriously doubt he ever slept in a tent in his entire life. But as philosophers, critical thinkers and ethical men, Mike and my father had a lot in common.

Mike once scolded my mother, kindly but firmly, after she recalled a practical joke she and Durant had played on my father ages before, not long after they were married. Durant was the mastermind, of course, but my mother participated. My father was a serious worrywart, a propensity Durant found entertaining. So they composed a telegram that went something like this: Help, help! House has burned down. Car has rolled off cliff. Dog has drowned. Roof has blown off school. Diptheria epidemic. Both legs broken. Tom and Ellie's bags packed, coming to live with you.

And they sent it to my father, who didn't get the joke. He took it seriously. He was alarmed and upset and angry. It threw his household into a panic.

"That wasn't funny, Mary," Mike said to my mother.

She protested. The "disasters" itemized in the telegram were so outlandish no one could have believed them. It was so obviously a joke!

"Maybe so," said Mike. "But it wasn't funny."

Occasionally the fog lifted from my mother's mind and she made perfect, lucid sense, saw things exactly as they were, and spoke the clear truth. "Oh, Ellie," she said once when she'd been with me for many months and our struggles were a vortex pulling us in, "I know I wouldn't have got old so quick if Mike hadn't died. When I think of what old age could have been . . ."

And so it was that I chugged a bottle of wine as fast as I could get the cork out on the evening of the day we took my mother to the Hostel. After the geriatrically early dinner, we'd walked her down the hall to her room. "We have to go on a trip, Mom," we said. "Out of town for a few days. You can relax here and not worry about anything. Let these nice folks take care of you while we're gone."

Oh, God. The look on her face when she comprehended that we were leaving her there. So many people who try to take care of someone with dementia talk about the suspicion, the paranoia, the accusations of malfeasance. My mother was never like that with me. She trusted me, even at her saddest, sickest, most confused. It had been a cinch to get her into the car, to go for a ride, to lead her down the hall after dinner. *She trusted me.* And there's the pain that I cannot beat to death, bury, burn, wall up or drown no matter how many gallons of Chardonnay I submerge it in or how long I hold it under.

Alcohol addles the brain, as we all know. But not right away. Sometimes when you're freshly intoxicated you can find yourself in a state of heightened lucidity. If I were a pianist, I would have sat down at the keys that night and made the house shake. My computer beckoned. Now, there was a keyboard I could play passably well. I drained my glass and flexed my fingers. Miss Wood would be proud.

You can't live with it, I wrote. Take it from me: Don't try. It will twist your love around and make you ill. Consider this a warning. You can't do it. I wish someone had warned me . . .

I'd be playing that little keyboard a lot over the next month. There was nothing else I could do.

March: I feel like one of those guys on a doomed Antarctic expedition, the last one alive, writing in his diary right up to the bitter end. Maybe somebody will find this alongside my frozen corpse.

My mother's been in the Hostel for a little over three weeks. The day after we took her there, she cried and begged to come home. The next few days were not so bad. I escorted her in to dinner on one of those nights and sat her down with the other old ladies at her table. They smiled and greeted her. I allowed myself a scrap of hope. People! Company! Attention! They all said it might be rocky at first, but that she'd adjust.

A day or so later, a fax from Jill, the head of the place: Your mother has been seriously agitated. We've put her on medication. Fine, I think, fighting back the alarm. Whatever it takes. Maybe that'll do it.

Next day, I go to visit. She's got her hat and coat on, and she's packed her clothes and toiletries into plastic bags and pillowcases. I want to come and try living with you, she says. No memory at all of the past sixteen months. I unpack her stuff while she cries and begs. Why can't I live with you? I'm all alone here, she says. All alone.

Calls at night: Announces she'll be "checking out" and going back to Connecticut to live with Joan Talbridge. The newspapers, she says, have reported that she's moving to California, but she's not. She's decided against it.

The next few days are a little better. A whole day goes by without any word from either her or the staff. My dreams and my sleep improve a little. I call her one afternoon, and Jill answers the phone in my mother's room. She's a little over-medicated, Jill says. I'm staying with her so she doesn't hurt herself. Whatever you need to do, I tell her, my heart flop-flipping like a toad in a jar, tacitly letting her know I'm not the litigious sort. Later, my answering machine flashing and flashing and flashing: ten messages from my mother. I'm all alone. I came all the way out here to visit you, and I'm stuck alone in this place. Oh, El-Belle! Where are you? Please, please call me.

Next time I see my mother, she's quite good. Calm, lucid, more or less coherent.

Then, whammo: A call from Jill. Your mother attacked the night person on duty so that he (!) had to go hide behind a door. Was smoking in her room. Was out on her deck, banging on the railing, screaming ELLIE! ELLIE! ELLIE! Waking up everyone. Her medication adjusted again.

A few more days when things seem to be improving. Then, one morning while I'm visiting, Jill takes me aside, says she needs to talk business.

Your mother, she tells me, is the most high-maintenance person here (read: biggest pain in the ass). If she's going to stay, you're going to have to hire private-duty help, or come and fill in yourself. She's wearing out the staff.

And here's the part that I kind of knew was coming, that maybe I've known was coming all my life:

She's frightening some of the other residents.

I'll sign off now. I've eaten the last of the sled dogs and the wind is howling so that my lantern's flickering and the walls of the tent are about to blow down. I'm running out of lamp oil anyway. I'll just roll up in my sleeping bag and wait for morning, if it comes. I'll consult the image of my mother when she was in her prime. Mom, am I doing the right thing? What would you do?

CHAPTER ELEVEN

Shiva, the Destroyer

Friday, March 31: a day that will live in infamy. I look back down the corridor of months to that afternoon: It's like watching myself in a jerky, grainy old home movie pieced together from fragments. I feel pity in a superior sort of way, the way we, the alive and well, can feel when we look at a smiling photograph of someone who was murdered or who died in a car crash. Ah, yes. There I was, climbing a ladder, carrying a bucket of paint and a brush. Am I waving at the camera? Poor innocent fool.

It was hot, the sky brilliant. That fact right there should have warned me that something was off; it never gets really hot here on this coast, not even in the middle of summer. Now, of course, I know where that heat came from. It was because the gods, sadistic little fat freckle-faced Gary Larson kids, had me under their magnifying glass.

My mother had been at the Hostel for about five weeks. Those five weeks had sure enough been payback time. When I was fourteen, I went off to boarding school and instantly loathed it. I plagued my mother with horrible weeping howling collect phone calls, every day, begging her to get me out of there. I was a colossal pain in the ass. She tried a little tough love for a while, but I was tougher, and kept up the squawking and kicking and crying with grim determination until Christmas vacation, when I came home and never went back to that school. I'd worn her down.

Yes. This was payback, with majorly compounded interest and penalties. By week four, my mother had everyone pretty well traumatized. Three different doctors were prescribing drugs with terrible-sounding names that made me think of evil warlords of enemy planets: Zyprexa, Thiothixene, Depakote, Risperdal. Darthvader. The red light on my answering machine, blinking and blinking and blinking frantic S.O.S.'s, looked to me like the eye of Lucifer himself in the darkness of my study. I'd listen, full of dread, finger poised over the fast-forward button, volume down as far as it would go so that I couldn't decipher her actual words and to minimize for my ears the unbearable anguish and confusion in her voice.

By Week Five, the final week in March, the administrator said my mother was officially on probation. By then I was buying the kind of wine that comes in a box with a little spigot. I was definitely going for quantity over quality; and the cheap sour taste, bad sleep and queasy hangovers seemed like appropriate punishment.

We came up with an idea: Send her to the Adult Activities Program at the senior center in the next town. The program I'd rejected because I would have had to have her ready to go by 8:30 A.M. But now she was at the Hostel, where being up and dressed and fed by 8:30 was a way of life.

Suddenly that feeble stupid senior center program was looking damned good. Retarded people eating Jell-O? Just the ticket. It was cheap, she'd get a nice lunch, she'd get a longish bus ride twice a day, she'd get out of the Hostel. Most important, they'd be rid of her for a good part of the day five days a week. She'd be dropped off around 3:00 in the afternoon, and then Allen would go up there and keep her out of trouble until about an hour after dinner. Maybe, just maybe, it would work.

Day One: With trepidation I call the Hostel that evening for a report. Surprise! Couldn't have gone better. Everyone delighted. Bus driver gallant with my mother. She eats a hearty dinner.

Day Two: Same as the day before. In addition to calling the Hostel, I call the director of the program, a chirpy cheery kindergarten teacher-sounding woman who says my mother's having a "wonderful" time, that everyone just "adores" her.

Day Three: I decide to butt out and not call either the Hostel or the program. No one calls me. Not even my mother. The phone is miraculously silent. No news, I reason, is good news.

Day Four: Same as Day Three. I relax by the smallest increment. Is that a ray of hope breaking through the clouds?

Day Five, Friday, March 31: Whistle while you work. Mitch and I undertake some long-postponed projects. We're busy little beavers. Aforementioned beautiful blazing blue day. I'm painting the front of the cottage, Mitch is fixing the car. Along about 2:00 a wee but adamant gnawing of guilt. Maybe . . . maybe I'll call the program, tell them not to put her on the bus, that I'll come get her myself and take her for a ride and then back to the Hostel. I have a vision of things normalizing.

I call. Someone asks if I can hold on for a moment. I hear murmuring, the scrape of a chair, a hand muffling the mouthpiece. Then the kindergarten woman gets on the phone. "Eleanor?" she says, and my viscera know before my ears hear.

My mother's been sent back to the Hostel early. Was sent back early yesterday as well. Why? Yesterday, because she'd left the building and couldn't be persuaded to return. And today because she started screaming and cursing in the middle of some kind of musical activity and hit one of the staff members, some woman who'd tried to pull her onto the "dance floor." Then she left the building again.

The kindergarten-teacher voice was deadly firm now, all traces of perkiness expunged. She read me a set of rules like a cop reading me my rights. My mother had committed the Big No-No: She'd hit someone. "We don't tolerate that behavior," said the women.

Heart in mouth, I call the Hostel. They're in a huge flap. You'd think my mother had bombed the place. No more slack for her. Expulsion is imminent. Suddenly the phrase "psych evaluation" is flying around like a little heat-seeking missile. The Hostel's own pill-dispensing shrink is the source. There's a geriatric psychiatric unit in Petaluma where he seems to think she should go right away.

Psych evaluation? Mitch and I don't know exactly what that means. We know what the individual words mean, of course, but we don't know what will actually happen to my mother if they put her through one. We consult Mitch's sister in Maryland. She's smart, compassionate, savvy, an RN, and she works inspecting nursing homes, just as Mitch once did. She says a psych evaluation is a necessity for the proper diagnosis and care of anyone with dementia, that my mother should have had one a long time ago.

Okay, we think. Maybe this is a piece of good luck. We've been floundering and flailing ever since she got here a year and a half ago. What the hell do we really know? The only thing we know for a fact is that she's been drugged into zombiehood. Her poor injured brain is marinating in a hissing, sparking pharmaceutical brew. She's slurring her words, stumbling, talking crazy talk. One of the more sympathetic staff people at the Hostel had whispered to me that she thought my mother's combative behavior was the drugs talking. "I've seen it before," she said: "I know when it comes from the person and when it comes from the drugs."

The psych evaluation means ten days in the hospital. I think: All right. They'll clean her up. They'll detox her, get her off all these medications, test her, find out what's really going on with her. Maybe they'll even figure out what's wrong with her stomach. A good thing, we tell ourselves. A good thing. But here's the naked truth: We'd sell our souls to avoid bringing her back home.

We call the psych unit. She can't be admitted until Monday at the earliest. The Hostel says they'll allow her to stay where she is over the weekend. Many calls back and forth between us, the hospital, the Hostel.

The name of another establishment emerges from the crazed cacophony of phone calls that afternoon: The Pines. A skilled nursing facility in Petaluma that specializes in dementia. Skilled nursing facility? Our ears perk up. This is what her long-term care insurance policy is supposed to pay for. We call the place. We talk to Shelley, the woman in charge of admissions. We tell her my mother will be in the geriatric-psych unit at the hospital in Petaluma for ten days. Shelley says we're in luck; they happen to have a vacancy. And more luck: The guy who does evaluations of prospective residents for The Pines happens to be vacationing up in our neighborhood, diving for abalone. Shelley calls him on his cell phone, he calls us and we arrange to meet at the Hostel the next day where he will see my mother. We call Shelley and tell her contact has been made. Shelley and the psych unit talk directly to each other, then she calls us back and tells us they've negotiated an arrangement by which my mother can be discharged directly to The Pines after the ten days in the hospital. Provided, of course, that she passes muster with the abalone-diver evaluator guy tomorrow.

Then we get down to the real business: The Pines, Shelley tells us in a practiced delivery which she's no doubt worked hard to perfect, costs $195 a day. My mother's insurance might possibly cover $125 of that; the rest will have to come out of her pocket. I do the math on the calculator while we're talking, then do it again thinking I've surely made a mistake. Nope; no mistake: the out-of-pocket amount comes to $2170 a month, almost exactly the monthly cost of the Hostel, on top of what the insurance might or might not pay. Total monthly fee $6045. Plus they require a $5000 deposit up front, and we will have to start paying the $195 a day immediately—a "bed hold" while she's in the psych unit. Numbers spiral to dizzying heights. That's an almost $7000 reservation fee. It's the lottery in reverse.

It's amazing what you can adjust to, though, and how fast. The prices pummel us about the head, shoulders and solar plexus, but we rise from the mat like Rocky in the fourteenth round. We call my brother in Colorado and tell him the news and give him the numbers. He takes it calmly, philosophically. Now he's braced and ready.

The Pines. The name exudes reassurance. I've formed a picture in my head of what it looks like. At $195 a day, it can only be a haven of beauty and tranquility. Restful. Leaves rustling, rolling lawns, maybe the sound of a fountain splashing. Birds twittering. Rose gardens. Yes! Rose gardens! I have a vision of a converted estate. I speak to Shelley one last time. "It's nice, right?" I ask her.

"Oh, it's a real special place," Shelley says. "It has a gorgeous view. It's way up on a hill. You're up above everything. I'm sitting in my office right now and I can just about see the whole town. And we have nice big trees. Pines." By the time we're finished talking, I'm ready to check in myself.

It's about 5:00 P.M. by now, only three hours or so since my fateful call to the Adult Activities Program, and we've gone from the shock of discovery to chaos and despair to what's starting to shape up as a viable, if staggeringly costly, arrangement. The mysterious serendipity mechanism of the universe seems to have engaged its gears. Things are falling into place like a film of a demolition run backward.

There's nothing to be done for the moment. Everything's in suspension until tomorrow. The psych unit will call us on Monday. Mitch mixes a pitcher of martinis. Ice and glass clink, a siren song.

We have a shotgun. It's loaded, the safety on. We keep it around for when the Manson family comes calling. With a shotgun, you don't exactly have to be an ace marksman. But probably you'll never even have to fire it, Mitch has told me. Just cock it. It's the ultimate businesslike sound, one that even the most crazed psycho will recognize when he hears it coming from the dark at the top of the stairs.

It's almost midnight, seven hours since we took our first sip of martini. I lie alone in the blackness in the loft on the old futon we drag out for guests. The shotgun is about three feet away from me. I'm giving serious consideration to using it on myself.

When I was very young, I used to ponder the riddle of how thought becomes will and will becomes action. I could sit there and think and think with all my might about picking up that pencil, but my hand was not going to move until thought was somehow translated into will. And I'd dissect the process into its smallest components, trying to pin down the exact moment of transition from thought to action. I never could.

So I lie in the dark thinking about picking up the shotgun, but my arms and legs don't get me up off the futon and over to where it is. Though I imagine every aspect: the noise, the mess, the driveway full of cop cars and ambulances and fire engines and whirling red and blue lights and the neighbors in their bathrobes. The white-sheeted gurney coming out the front door.

I know what a shotgun does at close range. I have a book downstairs, an L.A. homicide detective's personal scrapbook of photos called Death Scenes. There's an entire section devoted to shotgun suicides. Usually the head ceases to resemble a head in any way; it looks like exploded hamburger, the walls and ceiling dripping blood, bone and brains. I think about

Colonel Samsonoff. The talk was all over town about how they'd had to scrape the pieces from the ceiling. And that was just a rifle.

And I wonder how it is when your head is flying apart. Is there time for you to hear the huge roar of the shotgun? At what exact point is consciousness extinguished? I think: This is completely within the realm of possibility. The gun is right there. I could change everything for everybody forever, abruptly and decisively. With just a few small simple motions of my limbs and fingers, the slightest little adjustment in trajectory, I could swerve this procession right off the road and over the cliff. Take a little detour. People do it all the time. All the time. And I know: At the precise moment that I lie there thinking about it, dozens, maybe hundreds, of people on the planet, people with more resolution than I, have shotguns in their mouths or under their chins and are pulling the triggers. It's simply a statistical fact.

I think about George Sondergard, mild-mannered insurance agent, carrying his rope, climbing the creaking stairs to his attic with deliberation. Choosing the beam, arranging the chair, stepping up onto it. Putting the rope around his neck, tightening it. Talk about resolution. I imagine the tableau my own dangling corpse would present. The homicide detective's book has plenty of pictures of hangings, too, so I have a pretty good idea. How do you suppose Mitch would like that?

We fought that night. It started about an hour into our first pitcher of martinis. I can't tell you the details. Not because I don't remember. Au contraire; I remember every moment with perfect clarity. It's that I can't. Don't get me wrong. I'd love to tell you. I'm dying to tell you. It belongs in this story, and I could tell it so well. It's the kind of stuff writers kill to sink their fangs into. But I can't. Not now. Ask me about it in ten years—no, twenty—but not now. For now, it'll have to be enough for you to know that we fought, and it went on for hours and hours, and that by the time it ended I was a quivering blob of protoplasm contemplating extinction.

I will tell you this much: If I had used the shotgun on myself, one round would have more than done the job. But the forensic investigator examining the gun would have discovered that it had been fired twice that night.

My head reverberates with terrible echoes and lurid images of our desperate battle. After a very long time a weird calm descends, and with a bit of chemical assistance, I slip over some precipice into oblivion.

It's another hot, blue gorgeous day. I am poisoned, ravaged, shell-shocked, trembling with exhaustion, skull pounding. Rise and shine: Today is the day I'm to meet the guy from The Pines so he can evaluate my mother. Mitch and I move about the kitchen, two grim silent strangers.

I'm at the Hostel at noon sharp. My mother, as usual, is nicely dressed. Drugged, demented—it doesn't matter. She still pulls it together with style. I sit with her and her tablemates for lunch. One of them, Anna May, is ninety-eight and so deaf you have to shout directly in her ear, but she's got all her marbles and a great sense of humor. The other, Toni, is pretty far gone mentally, but she's docile, tractable—unlike some people we know.

My mother is tragically glad to see me. Naturally, she has no memory of the Senior Center debacle, and no idea at all of my condition, which would have appalled her old intact self (as would, of course, her own condition). The Pines guy appears, slips into a chair and pulls it up to the table. He's young, a jock, obviously pumps iron. He's wearing a white polo shirt with "The Pines" embroidered over the left breast pocket. I wish his shirt were green, or red, or purple. This is just a little too close to the Men in White who come to take you away. After lunch, he offers his arm. A man offering my mother his arm is not something she can resist. It's what she waited for more than half her life, until Mike came along. She doesn't ask who he is or why he's there; she just takes his arm.

We go to her room. He asks her a few simple questions: day of the week, when she was born, where she was born. She gets the last two right. He asks her to walk unassisted across the room. He feels her hands. Checking for what—temperature? Tremors? He's good at what he does, though. He's kind and respectful. I wonder how good he is at imagining what she once was. Not very, I'm pretty damned sure.

Then he and I go and sit on the deck outside the main door and talk. My bones ache. Little waves of sickness ripple the lining of my stomach at rhythmic intervals. There are flowers, hummingbirds, the blue sky, blooming rhododendron bushes, the woods all around. He says The Pines will take her. I ask him the same question I asked Shelley: Is the place . . . nice?

"Well," he says, looking around, "nothing could be as beautiful as this."

Monday: A friend lends us his large comfortable car for the ride to Petaluma. We go to the Hostel to pick up my mother. Despite the fact that she's stumbling and mumbling incoherently, she's all nicely dressed in a silk scarf and a white sweater, as if we're off on some fun expedition. Can my heart break any further?

They can't wait to be rid of her. They hand us a couple of bulging plastic bags of medications, enough to bring down an elephant. I look at the labels: Not only are there three different prescribing doctors, and at least five different medications, but we can see that the pills have been dispensed carelessly, because one of the medications, something called Depakote, comes in a big daily punch-out card like an Advent calendar. There are two of these cards, identical, each representing a month's supply of the same drug. One of them has had seven days' worth punched out and the other one has one day's worth punched out. Plainly, the meds have not been dispensed with the greatest of competence and attention. I draw your attention to exhibit number three, Your Honor.

We pack a suitcase for my mother. Jill hands me my mother's official eviction letter: thirty days' notice, an efficient summary of her less-than-satisfactory behavior since the day she arrived there—as if I needed it—plus details of more fun and games over the weekend since the incidents at the daycare program: wandering in the hall in her underwear with a lit cigarette, shouting, barging into other peoples' rooms, etc. Jill looks unhappy, eyes averted, when she hands me the letter. I feel sorry for her. I'd rather work in a rendering plant than have her job.

On the two-and-a-half-hour drive down, my drugged mother rides in the back seat. She mutters and drifts in and out. She doesn't ask where we're going or why. She's oblivious to the glorious spring all around us.

Same thing when we arrive at the hospital. Petaluma's a little city just south of Santa Rosa, more like a big town, parts of it attractive, other parts perfectly nondescript or downright ugly. It's in the vast Highway

101 corridor of suburbia and shopping malls that goes all the way from Santa Rosa to San Francisco and hundreds of miles beyond. But it's pretty civilized, Petaluma, human-scaled. The hospital is smallish, no more than three stories high, nice landscaping. None of that sprawling scary chaos you find in big-city hospitals. A pleasant friendly lady gives us directions to the geriatric-psych unit: Take that elevator, go to the top floor, take a left. You'll see the sign.

When we get there, we find a big set of locked stainless-steel double doors. We have to ring a bell to get in. A smiling nurse opens the door, greets us. Behind her is a decrepit ancient man strapped in a seat with an attached tray, like a full-sized highchair, food on the tray, chin on his chest. Not what I would have wished for as our first sight.

She'll have her own room and bathroom, at least, though it's distinctly a hospital room. They inventory her belongings. No sharp objects (nail scissors, tweezers, etc.) allowed. No scarves, handkerchiefs, belts. They make her take off her gold pin, a handsome plain rectangle she's particularly fond of, which she'd put on the front of her white sweater that morning thinking we were going somewhere pleasant.

I have my power-of-attorney papers with me. My mother signed them willingly, trustingly, a couple of years before. There's her big loopy signature. I sit at the desk and fill out reams of forms and answer questions. I tell the nurse about the overmedicating, the chronic upset stomach, the years of despair and depression and vodka martinis after Mike's death. I try to cram as much useful information into the interview as I possibly can so that maybe they can actually help her. Then it's time to go. I tell her I'll call that night, that I'll call every day. She's totally desolate, no idea at all of where she is or why. Yes, my heart can break further. The big doors slam and lock behind us.

In the car, we decide maybe we'd better go have a look at The Pines before we start giving them almost $200 a day plus a $5000 deposit and then hand my mother over to them, sight unseen.

As soon as we pull into the parking lot I've rejected the place. It's up on a hill, all right, just as Shelley promised, with a panoramic view of Petaluma and beyond, but that's not quite the same thing as a panoramic view of, say, Florence, or even Buffalo, New York. What you see are endless acres of freeways and shopping centers. Better no view than this view.

And yes, there are some okay trees, the eponymous "pines," but we're looking at a low, flat hospital building, probably 1950s vintage. Dismal yellowish stucco. Chain-link fence. My converted estate with the rose garden goes staticky and vanishes.

Inside, it's fluorescent lighting and linoleum floors. Pure, 100 percent institution. We meet Shelley. You'd think that eventually we'd learn that voices over telephones invariably produce pictures in our minds of strictly fictional characters. Shelley resembles my mental picture of her even less than The Pines resembles my fantasy estate. Her voice had conjured a plump-but-solid middle-aged woman with dark curly hair. Instead we find ourselves shaking hands with a skeletal little blonde with long wispy hair who looks about fourteen. She has to be a speed freak, I think, estimating her weight at maybe eighty-three pounds. Her portrait would blend right in with the ones you see in the post office: MISSING CHILD. LAST SEEN 6/14/97. STRANGER ABDUCTION.

She shows us around. The famous urine smell you hear so much about is absent; instead, the place is redolent with industrial-strength disinfectant. There are advanced dementia people shuffling and wandering. One guy looks not much older than fifty and his legs are in a sort of rolling apparatus like those training devices they use with little kids just learning to walk. He wears red pajamas and lets loose with big guffaws of laughter from time to time.

When Mitch was inspecting nursing homes for the state, he got his most valuable information, he said, from the patients themselves. He'd approach anybody—they could be slumped in a wheelchair, drooling, eyes vacant, or lying on a bed, mouth open, corpse-like—so still he'd have to watch the bedclothes for a moment for signs of respiration—no matter. He'd walk right up, put a friendly hand on an arm or a shoulder and say, "Hello, how are you, I'm Mitch, what's your name?" He didn't always get an answer, but he said you'd be amazed at how often he did. And then he'd ask (loudly), "ARE YOU GETTING ENOUGH TO EAT? HOW ARE THEY TREATING YOU?"

Today, at The Pines, he swings into action. I'm impressed. It's the look of surprise on peoples' faces that you notice first. Eh? What? Someone's talking to me? And for a moment, some of them come back from far, far away.

There's a dayroom with big windows and jolly colorful idiotic pictures on the walls. Mitch stops and has a conversation with a woman who's sitting in the room with her husband, whom she placed here only a couple of weeks before. She's drowning in guilt. She tells Mitch she's been there every day since he was admitted, and she's thinking about taking him out. The husband, a big, strongly built man with enormous leathery hands, who obviously did hard physical work all his life, is silent. Stares out the window at the scrubby woods and a power pole.

I can't wait to get out of there. Even though we've barely said a word, Shelley knows the score. Like any salesperson, she sees when the prospect has slipped irrevocably away and knows when to quit wasting her energy. We thank her for meeting us, ask for a copy of their latest state inspection report, and split.

Out the door, we look at each other and agree: No way. No fucking way. Even if it cost ten cents a day. Even if they paid US. I'd rather show my mother an open grave.

The guilty wife back at The Pines had mentioned another place: Adobe House. "It's beautiful," she'd said. "But too expensive." I wonder how it could be more expensive than The Pines. We find it after dark. It's a big faux hacienda-type building, so common in California, in the middle of a shopping-mall neighborhood. Even though we've arrived unannounced, a housekeeper lets us in. The urine smell hits us in the face even out in the tastefully appointed lobby. In the twilit halls around a big central courtyard, it's a Night of the Living Dead promenade. One old guy paces in long johns and a bulging diaper. Another fellow, jaunty and grinning, wearing a Tyrolean hat with a feather, greets us merrily. I honestly can't tell if he's a visitor or an inmate. All that's missing is crazy carnival music. We thank the housekeeper, grab a glossy brochure just to be polite, and beat it the hell out of there, too.

We're beginning to get the picture. Wherever we put her, she'll be in hell. And so will I.

CHAPTER TWELVE

Hungry Ghosts

I call her at the hospital every day. Sometimes she's almost coherent. Mostly she's so far out there I can't even guess what she's trying to say. Her electronic voice is tiny and distant. All I can do is enunciate desperate useless words into the telephone while she slips into another dimension, like talking in a dream, like losing radio contact with someone drifting into outer space. Conversations with the staff are even less encouraging. We hear of crying, fits, tantrums.

We drive down to visit her exactly one week into her stay. We called ahead to tell them we're coming, and they warned us that she'd be wearing a sort of restraint vest. They make it sound like the most innocent version of such a garment. A "posey" vest, they call it. It's just to keep her from hurting herself, they say. Her first night there, apparently, she got up to pee, leaked a little on the linoleum floor, slipped and fell and cut her hand. And she's "restless," as they put it. Gee, I think; if only I had a "posey" vest to wear with my new bonnet and gloves, I could be the grandest lady in the Easter parade. Dread congeals around me the closer we get to the hospital.

We are ushered into a side room set up for families and visitors. Coffee machine, dreary sofas, *Reader's Digest* and *Popular Mechanics* on a table. We'll confer with the psychologist before we visit my mother.

Remember William Macy's car salesman in *Fargo*? It took me a while to recognize him out of context, but there he was in the person of the psychologist—big fakely sincere anxious watery eyes, lopsided grin, talking a streak of slippery blarney designed to divert us and hypnotize us so we won't notice that he's essentially saying nothing at all.

He flips through her already amazingly thick medical charts, letting us see bits and pieces but keeping a firm grip on it. He's determined that we not actually hold it in our hands. Mitch especially knows that this is not legal. Families have every right to see medical records, but we tacitly agree that it would be impolitic to make a scene. He blathers on about medications, psychological tests, blood tests, EKGs, but it quickly becomes evident that their main business is to tinker with her multiple medications, scarcely cleaning her up the way I thought they would. They are simply doing their job: Fine-tuning her to be an ideal sedated nursing home candidate, a consumer of costly drugs.

An attendant comes in, says Mary has heard our voices and wants to see us. They bring her in. Take another little piece of my heart. The vest, which actually has a cute decorative pattern on it, cavorting lambs or bunnies or some fucking thing like that, has long dangling and very serious-looking canvas straps. The chains on Marley's ghost. A nurse is holding my mother up; when she sees me, she forcefully shrugs the woman's hand from her arm and says, "Let GO of me!" She hugs me as if she hasn't seen me for ten years. Mitch, too.

The shrink and the nurse can't get out of there fast enough. We're alone with my mother. We sit there on the Naugahyde sofas. Her hand is bandaged from her fall. Her eyes are red-rimmed, inflamed, struggling to focus. She fiddles with the canvas straps. She looks at us from another planet. We try to explain why she is there, why she can't leave with us that day, but the truth is, we don't know the answers to those questions. We know we are no different from the other dissembling morons who've been holding her prisoner for a week. There is a stupid destructive pointlessness to the entire proceeding that's been starkly revealed so that it's impossible to ignore, hide or rationalize.

Years ago, I went to the Dublin Zoo, reputed to be one of the best in the world. The animals supposedly lived in "natural" habitats and were much happier than other zoo animals. I remember standing on one side of a moat which separated me from the orangutan habitat. The moat was not very wide, maybe fifteen feet, but apparently that was enough because orangutans hate water and the moat was as effective as a set of steel bars. One big scruffy male squatted at the water's edge on the other side of the moat and looked directly into my eyes. What I saw in those eyes, which are virtually human, was unambiguous. I knew what he was seeing: another ape of some sort. An enemy ape who was free while he was not. He knew he was a prisoner, and what I saw in his eyes was pure psychotic hatred. What I saw in my mother's eyes that day was not so different; just substitute betrayal, bewilderment and bitterness for hatred. Drugged, crazy, abandoned and tortured, my mother still could not hate me. She still loved me, and I was unworthy of that love. I felt like the lowest piece of shit on earth. She was fighting, fighting, through the chemicals, like someone in a hypnogogic state who can't quite come out of a dream, trying to make sense of it, but talking crazy talk at the same time.

"These people here," she says, sotto voce. "They're actors. Arthur Miller owns this place."

"Wuh?" is all I can think of to say, a fresh new panic I'd not felt before washing through me.

Yet even through the swimming kaleidoscope of her consciousness she's trying, trying to understand. She's still in there somewhere, and she's not giving up. And we have nothing at all to offer her except to tell her we'll get her out, at the end of the week, before much more torture is inflicted on her.

We leave. We drive on the freeway, dazed, silent. There is no other word for what we've just seen except abuse. What have we done? For Christ's sweet sake—what have we done? Bring her out to California and make her happy, eh? Well, you're certainly doing a brilliant job. A brilliant job. I've never felt so ill with misery and guilt. I would be glad to self-destruct, just vanish in a cloud of acrid smoke.

Right there in the car, Mitch and I break the vow we made to each other when we put her in the Hostel a little over a month before—that no matter what, we won't bring her back to live with us. Temporarily, of course, we tell each other. Until we find a solution.

★ ★ ★

My mother's mother lived to almost ninety without dementia or seri-ous health problems. She just got old. Too old to go on living in her lit-tle apartment in New York. So my mother moved her up to Connecticut when my grandmother was about eighty-two.

She stayed with my mother and Mike in their house for a while, and then my mother moved her to an old folks' boardinghouse ten minutes away. This was before the term "assisted living" was a glimmer in any-one's eye. This place wasn't even an official "rest home." I doubt if the woman who ran it had any sort of license or training; she was just a country widow with a big roomy ramshackle Victorian house. She did all the work and cooked all the meals for about four oldsters at a time, and that's how she supported herself and her kids. I never knew what the rate was, but I'll bet it wasn't any twenty-three hundred a month or its equivalent in 1970s dollars.

My mother moved my grandmother because she and Mike agreed that it wouldn't work to have her living right there in their house with them. And it wasn't because my grandmother was a bitch or hard to handle or needed help walking or dressing. She was a sweet, tractable person, self-effacing to a fault, reasonable and undemanding. She had arthritis, but she walked pretty well with her cane. She could climb stairs. She took care of her own grooming, bathing, dressing. Even so, her presence put a strain on things, as my mother and Mike knew it would. The plan had been, right from the moment of moving her out of New York, that her stay with them would be temporary. She was there for maybe a month, maybe two.

When the time came to move to the boarding house, my grand-mother didn't want to go. She wanted to stay with my mother and Mike. Who could blame her? It was a big house. Mike was jovial and flirty with her. There were evening cocktails (my grandmother's drink watered way down), pleasant dinners, company, the bosom of the family. But my mother and Mike were firm in their resolve, and the move was made.

The boardinghouse was perhaps not without flaw. She had her little complaints. My grandmother was one of the last of the Victorian gen-tleladies—well-traveled, refined, Vassar Class of 1911—and a few aspects of her new home didn't quite meet her standards, like the senile tooth-less guy who wore a plastic bib at the table ("Should have been dead long ago," was my grandmother's comment) or the old, old, old lady well past her hundredth birthday, mostly blind and deaf, who spent all her time in bed making demands in her foghorn voice. The woman who ran the house had kids, a couple of rambunctious pre-teen boys, and my grandmother claimed that the older one occasionally exposed himself to her.

But she adjusted. A big help in that department was the fact that the town where my mother lived was where my grandmother had spent her summers for years and years when my mother was growing up, and so she had plenty of friends and acquaintances, some of them going back fifty years. They came and took her to church and to lunch and to the movies and for nice rides around the lake. She was back in her old stomping grounds. And every week or so, my mother and Mike had her over to dinner. When they traveled, which they did a lot during the seventies for the Audubon book, they knew she was getting plenty of attention and care and was never lonely.

She lived there for almost eight years. She was in excellent health virtually right up to the moment she died. She never had surgery of any kind in her entire life. (When she moved out of New York, it was dis-covered that she hadn't been to a doctor since my mother was born in 1922.) She spent only about twelve hours in the hospital on the night of her death from a sudden, massive and very decisive stroke. She made it well into her ninetieth year without nursing homes, lingering money-draining illnesses, senility, pain, loss of dignity, loneliness.

She'd had her share of heartache—forced by her family to marry a man she didn't love (my grandfather), a baby son (before my mother) dead of Sudden Infant Death Syndrome (she was the one who went to pick him up after his nap, found him limp and lifeless), divorce, a second marriage when she was in her sixties to a terrific guy (I remember him) who went and dropped dead a couple of months after the wedding. But she had a wonderful equanimity. She dried her tears, and the next twenty-five years of her life were pleasant, right up to the last day.

I was young and stupid, and thought this was standard procedure. You live to be really old without any serious problems, surrounded by lifelong pals and family, and then you die neatly, quickly, cleanly.

I've been, as they say, disabused.

We could have taken my mother back to the Hostel after the hospital. She was only ten days into her thirty-day notice. They would have had to take her for the rest of the month, which was already paid for. It's a measure of my guilt and horror—and more impressively, of Mitch's— that we nix the idea and decide to bring her directly home.

In a spasm of remorse, we clean and fix and paint in the cottage. Finish things we never finished. Spruce and freshen it up, put a coat of gorgeous red paint on the double front doors. Prepare it for a big Welcome Home. I've heard that childbirth is hideously painful, that women have been known to swear they'll never do it again, but then some sort of amnesia hormone kicks in and they do it again. Remorse, I have learned, is a thousand times more powerful than any hormone.

Not even a month and a half since the day we tricked my mother into the Hostel, I'm emptying her room there. And such a pleasant room it is. Airy, comfortable, carpeted. A magnificent bathroom. A private deck. A magnolia tree with big pink blossoms standing over it, dropping its luxuriant petals.

A short drive from my house. Almost the same distance as from my grandmother's boardinghouse to my mother and Mike's house. To think that I had actually entertained visions of having my mother over to dinner, taking her to the movies . . .

It's gloomy, chilly, spatters of rain. I pack all her stuff into the car in one load. Jill, still avoiding eye contact, gives me a refund check. Hands me two remaining bottles of fake wine. I try for a little levity: If only this were real, I say.

Not that it matters that it isn't; my flask of vodka is under the seat in the car. I'm pretty sure Jill could smell the fumes emanating from me. But I don't care.

★   ★   ★

I have a recent photograph I keep in a drawer. Every once in a while, when I'm in the mood for a little self-loathing, I take it out and look at it. It's a picture of me, my mother and an old family friend, Augusta. The friend is my age, and is in fact the daughter of Joan, the woman my mother always talked about going to live with back in Connecticut. Out of range of the camera, Joan is watching while Mitch takes the picture. Joan is the exact same age (seventy-seven then) as my mother. Her mind is perfectly intact. I am sick with jealousy.

In the picture, Augusta, my mother and I are standing in front of a Petaluma restaurant's outdoor mural, a vivid undersea scene. We're about to go in and have lunch. My mother is holding on to my arm, her head turned slightly, looking at the camera. She has a vague little smile on her face, and around her eyes is an expression as if someone's talking to her in Swahili. Augusta's expression is complicated. There's alarm, philosophic detachment and humor on her face all at the same time. My own face, caught in the act of talking, cracking some joke, looks to my merciless eye the way it did when I tripped on LSD years ago and stood in front of a mirror (advice: not for the faint of heart): clownish, mendacious, distorted. Since I recall exactly what I was thinking when the picture was taken, I can read that face like a geologist reading a topographical map. I know what's underneath. Someone else looking at the picture might be fooled into thinking this was a worthy person, a competent, dependable, compassionate person, somebody who would take good care of her ill, needy mother. But I'm not fooled. I know the truth. I look at the picture and think: *You phony. You liar. You rotten deceitful useless loveless craven weak selfish sack of shit.* Then I look at my mother's face again, see how she holds my arm for protection. *She trusts you.* Then I go back to my own face. And so on.

That picture was taken the day we got my mother out of the hospital after her "psych evaluation." Joan happened to be in San Francisco visiting Augusta, and had called the week before to ask if they could come for a visit. She didn't know about the expulsion from the Hostel, the drugging, the hospital. I told her the whole sorry sordid tale, and said I hated to have her see my mother in this condition, but she said,

I'm pretty tough, you know. True. Her husband had died a long lingering death, and she took care of him to the end.

Okay, then, I said, you and Augusta drive up and meet us in Petaluma on the day we spring her. We'll all go in together.

And we do. I'm glad they are there. It isn't just me and Mitch. And both of them, sturdy Yankees, are tough. They were like Anne Bancroft in *The Elephant Man,* when the great lady she plays meets him for the first time, and for just the smallest moment a temblor rolls across her features, about one-point-six on the Richter scale, then her face composes itself, she smiles radiantly and extends her hand as if he were the handsomest guy in the world.

Not that my mother is the Elephant Man. But neither Joan nor Augusta have seen her for a long time. It's been four or five years since Augusta has seen her, a year and a half for Joan. If they had seen her a mere couple of months ago, before the Hostel, before the drugging, before the hospital, they would have been in for perhaps a mild adjustment of expectations, but they would have been able to have a conversation with her. She still would have been able to pull it together.

But when we arrive to get her out of the hospital, my mother's been through the meat grinder. She's not as bad as when we were last down, but that's because they've stamped out the last of the little brush fires. They've found just the right drug combination to render her dazed and docile. Pharmaceutically vanquished, she's not fighting anymore.

For the entire year and a half that she'd been with us, scarcely a day went by without my mother speaking Joan's name. I could go live with Joan Talbridge. Joan invited me to come live with her. Maybe I should move in with Joan. You'd think that when she finally saw Joan, she'd fall all over her. But she just kind of smiles and says hello. I know she absolutely recognizes Joan's face, but I think the name floats around in one part of her fractured brain and the face in another.

The hospital staff try to give us some grief when we announce that we're taking her home and not to The Pines. The William Macy psychologist hems and haws to the effect that he'll be forced to put on her record that we removed her against medical advice. Mitch says that maybe the Medical Quality Board would like to hear about the "posey vest" and a few other things, like the fact that she was never detoxed. William Macy says he guesses it won't be necessary to put it on her record that we took her out against medical advice.

Then they hand us a sheaf of prescriptions that we're to fill. Some of the same evil warlords, plus a few new ones. "She really needs to have these medications professionally administered," they say, as if we'll then say, "Oh, okay, guess we'd better drop her off at The Pines after all." Our plan, of course, is to toss the prescriptions in the trash.

That's about the extent of our plans, except to go ahead and take her home and de-drug her. We don't have the remotest notion of what we'll do after that.

Her gold pin, the one she loved and was wearing the day she was checked into the hospital, is lost.

There's another photograph Mitch took that day. It was before we left the hospital. Joan and my mother are sitting in chairs, side by side. The fluorescent hospital lights are harsh. Joan is saying something to somebody standing nearby, so her face is upturned and her mouth is slightly open. The lights are making big shadows under her eyes. My mother has a tidy little smile. Her eyes look focused and wise. Her head is tilted so that it looks as if she's listening patiently, indulgently.

I imagine not knowing these two women and being shown this picture. And being told: One of them is drugged and demented and just spent ten days in the geriatric psych unit, where she cried and screamed and had to be tied down, but the other is eminently sane and whole and is visiting her unfortunate friend. Can you guess which is the damaged woman?

I'd look at the picture, consider for about a second, then point at Joan, and say, "It's obviously this one."

There's a nursing home in the town eight miles to the north of where we live. It's called Dunwood Oaks, though there are in fact no oaks there. Skilled nursing facilities or institutions specializing in Alzheimer's are where you go when you have the non-docile form of dementia, when you are beyond the scope of board-and-care or assisted living.

Trees or no trees, Dunwood Oaks is a skilled nursing facility. And though people groan and make faces when they hear the name, it isn't because it's so outstandingly horrible. It's just that it is what it is: a perfectly unglamorous small-town nursing home. I'd never considered it as even the remotest option.

During the two-and-a-half hour ride home from Petaluma, Mitch drives, my mother rides in the passenger seat and I'm in the rear. My mother asks perhaps seven or eight times for the name of the doctor she saw last time she was here, because, she says, her stomach is upset.

I can read the back of Mitch's head as if it were his face. By the time we pull into our driveway, I've decided that Dunwood Oaks will be my mother's next home.

CHAPTER THIRTEEN

Arsenic

She pushes open the door to her cottage and walks in. Everything's back where it was—typewriter on the desk, TV on the table with a bouquet of flowers on it, clothes in the closet and bureau drawer. The place sparkles. We've scrubbed the bathroom, the kitchen sink and the refrigerator, repainted the kitchen counter, mopped the floor, cleaned the rugs, vacuumed every square inch, washed the windows. It's been some serious penance. I actually spent a good long time on my knees. Mitch is optimistic that she'll be delighted and happy.

My mother puts her basket on the table as if she's been gone for maybe an hour. Polly strolls in, and in a classic display of feline demonstrativeness, also acts as if my mother's been gone for maybe an hour. Mom opens a can of cat food, feeds Polly, lights a cigarette, goes to the sink and fills a saucepan with water to make tea. She asks if we have enough food for her to have dinner with us tonight.

For me and Mitch, it's also seeming as if she never left. But the feeling is just a wee bit more complicated than it is for my mother and for the cat, two creatures who dwell in the eternal present. For us, it's like one of those time-and-space conundrums that physicists like to baffle and dazzle us regular mortals with. If you go fast enough—or is it slow enough?—a thousand years will be compressed into a few seconds!

That old conundrum must have got us. We know she's been gone for six and a half weeks. We lived every moment of that six and a half weeks, ricocheted around in its length, breadth, and depth, measured it with our whiskers so that its size and shape are imprinted indelibly on our internal calendars. But . . . it feels like about an hour.

That evening, I don't just lay out her breakfast stuff and wait until she's ready for bed and say goodnight the way I did for a year and a half. I'm going to stay with her in the cottage until she's asleep. She goes to bed; I sit on the couch in the other room and read. I won't leave until I hear snores. But little solar flares of anxiety have her up and down and in and out of bed over and over and over. "It's okay, Mom, I'm here, I'm here, it's okay, just go to sleep," I say. But it takes two Lorazepam and a couple of hours before I finally hear a snore and sneak out, shutting the door behind me with infinite care like someone in a movie defusing a bomb.

In the morning, her curtains are drawn and the cottage is silent long after I'm up. This is not the way it usually is.

It's another brilliant day. I've been thoroughly reconditioned: Bright blue days are ominous. Bad things happen beneath cheerful skies. That's how it is in this world. I walk across the driveway, the sun hot on my back. I'm under that magnifying glass. I think about all the other people on earth who are doing exactly what I'm doing at this exact moment.

I open the door to the cottage. Stillness.

Mom?

No answer.

These moments do arrive, I tell myself. They do. On gorgeous days just like this.

I creep into the bedroom. She's on her side, a pillow over her head, her arm crooked up alongside her face. I hold my breath like steadying a telescope. I watch the blankets.

After a long time, they rise, ever so gently. My mother is breathing.

We stop the drugs cold turkey, asking no medical advice. Rash? Maybe. But I know my mother's physical vitality. At the end of the first day home, she's already coming out of it. She has no memory of the Hostel or the psych unit, of course. No conscious memory, anyway. But her organism—every cell in her body—remembers, knows she's been keelhauled. She's a little shakier, a little clingier. She's definitely slipped a few notches. She was already damaged, and now she's been damaged more, and there is no way around the fact that I have been a party to putting her in harm's way.

She stops the shuffling and mumbling almost immediately, though the crazy talk pops out of her mouth occasionally for a couple of days more.

"Where's the old lady from Kent (Connecticut) who takes milk to old people?" she asks me one night when she's getting ready for bed. And: "When is the man coming who plays religious music on the piano?" My mother was a life-long and ardent nonbeliever who would fiercely chase Jehovah's Witnesses from her door. I once heard her ask an old gent with a sheaf of *Watchtowers* in his hand how he'd like it if SHE came to HIS house and tried to talk him into NOT believing in God.

Such talk tapers off and goes away. Rasputina again. What replaces it is amazingly lucid by comparison, though, of course, heart-ripping.

"I feel very badly," she says a few days after we bring her home. "Moving in on you and Mitch like this. I really should find a nice old folks' home."

We sigh.

"Actually, Mom," I say though I know I shouldn't, "we did find you just about the pleasantest old folks' home in the world. We'd move in there ourselves if we could. But they threw you out."

"Really? What did I do?"

"Well, you basically raised hell. Smoked in your room. Hit people. Yelled and screamed."

She laughs, gives me an incredulous look as if this were some great joke. "I don't remember any of this."

"Well, I do."

"Maybe we should try them again."

"Um—I don't think so, Mom."

"I should go back to Connecticut and live with Joan Talbridge."

"That's not such a great idea either."

"Why not?"

"She can't take care of you," I say tiredly.

"There's an old folks' home in New Preston [Connecticut]. I should go there."

"That place doesn't exist anymore, Mom."

"Well, I feel very badly, moving in on you and Mitch. It's not fair." Here's my opening.

"Well, uh, there is another place, actually, just up the road from here. We could check it out."

"I should go back to Connecticut and live with Joan Talbridge."

About five days after her return, she's standing on the front deck of our house. I'm in the bathroom, just getting out of the shower. Before I went into the shower, I told her where I was going and wrote a big note saying: MOM—I'M IN THE SHOWER AND WILL BE OUT IN 20 MIN- UTES! I showed it to her, left it on the dining room table. I'm naked, wrapping a towel around my head, when I hear my mother outside shouting my name, an edge of hysteria in her voice. I fling open the bathroom window.

"I'm HERE, for Christ's sake!"

"Oh, thank God," she says. "I didn't know where you were. I thought you'd left without me."

Mitch and I leave Allen with my mother one afternoon and go have a closer look at Dunwood Oaks. We don't call first, we just go. That's how you do it, Mitch says. Don't give them any warning.

It's dumpy and plain and hospital-like, but pretty lively, consider- ing what it is. The halls are noisy and something's going on every- where. It's almost pleasantly chaotic. There are the usual vacant-eyed corpses in wheelchairs here and there, but none of that awful tomb- and-doom quiet. An old lady resident wearing sequined blue denim and lots of mascara gloms onto us and takes it upon herself to give us a tour of the residential wing where she lives. The rooms are shared, but there's a college-dorm atmosphere—teddy bears and colorful blankets on the beds, pictures and knickknacks and posters on the walls. Mitch does what he always does—walks right up to people and asks them how they like the place. Another old lady, this one in a wheelchair in one of the dining rooms, takes hold of my arm while she tells us that she loves it, it's wonderful, everyone is so kind, she's so glad she's here, and on and on.

We are, in short, very pleasantly surprised indeed. My permanently knotted guts unclench a millimeter or two. Maybe the answer was right here under our noses all along. Maybe, just maybe, this could work. A big lively noisy place, which the Hostel certainly was not. And since it's a skilled nursing facility, her long-term care insurance would probably pay for it. And it's only a ten-minute ride from our house.

We're excited. We go to the office and put in our official application. Yes, small-town living has its pluses. But then there's the flip side of everyone knowing everyone else's business. Dunwood Oaks calls us a day or so later. It seems that they have already heard about my mother. The word's out. She's branded: combative. The scarlet letter. The big, bad No-No. And that's what they say to us after they make a few phone calls, including one to the daycare program: No. No.

Rejected by Dunwood Oaks? Can this be happening? Yes, it can. And thus it was that we wound up crawling on our knees in supplication to a place we once didn't deign to consider.

Not at first, though. Mitch swings into action. We won't take no for an answer, he says. We'll come back with counteroffers. Like doing a real-estate deal.

Mitch knows the laws and language. He also possesses an enviable fearlessness. He struck terror into many a greedy heart when he was an inspector of nursing homes, and he shut quite a few of them down. That's the kind of confrontation he thrives on and the mere thought of which turns my spleen to jelly.

This is no exception. He calls Dunwood Oaks back and arranges a special meeting with the guy who owns the place, the guy's daughter, who's the administrator, and the Big Head Nurse. He puts on a suit and tie, and Cary Grant-like, storms the place. Not to shut them down or intimidate them, but to negotiate, frankly, firmly and face-to-face. I, chickenheartedly, stay home.

They convene. Mitch says they shouldn't give a final answer until they've met my mother, see for themselves who it is they're rejecting. "She was overmedicated," he says. "She's detoxed now. She's a different person. And"—he adds this like sprinkling a little hot sauce into a stew—"Eleanor's mental health depends on this."

He gets them to agree to another meeting. It'll be the same personnel plus me and my mother. We go the very next day.

My mother is in fact de-drugged, and her manners are impeccable. My manners are impeccable, too, but I'd be lying if I said I was also de-drugged. Prince Valium was my escort.

Though we all make nice, it's a serious meeting. I'm dripping anxiety. The owner is a genuinely softhearted guy; I can see that right away. The head nurse is kind; after they've met my mother and chit-chatted a little, the nurse says: "C'mon, Mary; let's go look around." She takes my mother away so that we can get down to business.

The father defers to his daughter, who keeps her desk between her and us while he sits off to the side in a folding chair. It's plain that she is just about one hundred percent opposed to any compromise. She says that while they do have a great many residents with dementia, the facility is small and is not equipped to handle difficult or violent cases. "We have to think of the other residents," she says. "We have to think of the community as a whole. We just don't have the staff."

Mitch and I are pouring on the charm. See how reasonable and accommodating we are. What good listeners. Dad is susceptible, laughing at our little jokes, responding in a friendly way, but she's not buying it. She hangs very, very tough. I can tell that if it were up to Dad, he'd probably let my mother in. The daughter is the lion at the gate.

We make our offer: There's good reason to believe the drugs contributed to Mom's combative behavior. Give her ninety days. If it doesn't work, we'll take her out. We'll sign papers to that effect.

They say they'll think about it over the weekend, have another meeting on Monday, make a decision.

Meantime, I hear about a place in Davis, California, a skilled nursing facility with an Alzheimer's unit and an available "female bed." I make the drive on a Saturday. It takes four hours to get there. I stay about twenty minutes. I'm getting used to these places by now. Again, scarcely a snake-pit, but I instantly disdain the fluorescently lit institutional atmosphere and the never-never land shopping-mall neighborhood.

And the people in the Alzheimer's unit are way, way farther gone than my mother. Drooling, unable to speak. There's an open yard with a chain-link fence where they can wander. I thank the director politely and drive the four hours back to the coast through some of northern California's most staggeringly beautiful country—hills, vineyards, lakes, everything lush and velvety green from the spring rain, but I'm looking at it through dead eyes.

On Monday, they call from Dunwood Oaks to say they'll have their lawyer draw up papers to the effect that they'll take her only on a two-week-to-two-week trial basis, and we will have another meeting first.

Hallelujah, we think. Our foot's in the door. We'll make it work somehow. We arm ourselves, too, just to make sure. We do a little research in the *Physician's Desk Reference* on the various drugs the shrink back at the Hostel (who's also Dunwood Oaks' shrink) put her on, in particular an anti-psychotic that comes with an explicit warning that this medication should be used only with great caution on elderly women.

Mitch has a telephone conversation with the shrink, mentions this, makes it clear that he is to recommend my mother's admission to Dunwood Oaks. The shrink, perhaps sensing that there's the potential for a teensy bit of trouble, agrees to do that.

The place in Davis calls about an hour later, says someone else is interested in the bed, and do we want it or not? Thinking we've got Dunwood Oaks by the balls, only ten minutes away instead of four hours, I tell them no. The meeting at Dunwood Oaks is set for Tuesday.

On Tuesday, Dunwood Oaks calls and says their lawyer told them no such two-week agreement would be binding, and so the whole deal's off. We just can't risk a "catastrophic event," says the head nurse. I say darkly that there'll be a catastrophic event around our house any minute now.

But it's final: They will not take her. So: No Dunwood Oaks, and the place in Davis is lost.

The next day, the pharmacy bill for the huge bag of pills they handed me the day I picked up my mother at the Hostel arrives in the mail, run up during her four-week stay: six hundred and twelve dollars.

CHAPTER FOURTEEN

Old Lace

April:

"Can you hear the seals barking?"

"I think so."

"Listen. Hear that? That yelping? Those are seals on the buoy out in the bay. They crowd onto it, and other ones try to get on, and the ones that are already on block the ones trying to get on and they bark and bark. AHRT! AHRT! AHRT!"

"Isn't that extraordinary."

"Yeah. And I've seen 'em a couple of miles up the river. They swim up there where the fishing's good and there's less competition and no sharks."

"Mmmm-hmmmm."

"That's what I'd do if I were a seal. I'd stay the hell out of the ocean and go live in the river."

"All by yourself."

"The piano keys are too distant and there's the evaporation factor . . ."

What??

I jolt awake, startled by the strangeness of the dream-talk coming out of my own mouth. I'm lying on the grass next to my mother's lawn chair where she's stretched out. The sun blazes down. I have a low-grade fever. I'd flopped there and was chatting with her, wandering in and out of consciousness, luxuriating in the heat of fever and sun, and for a second or two slid down into delirium.

I have the flu. Mom, seventy-seven years old and a smoker, got a mere case of the sniffles while I came down with a raw, painful chest cold and a temperature. I can fall asleep standing up, sitting down, walking. My thousand and one responsibilities, obligations, anxieties recede into irrelevance. I just don't care. Flat on my back on the grass, the brilliant light penetrating my eyelids and my head pleasantly baking while peculiar sentences rise to my tongue, I have an insight: I think perhaps I've had a little glimpse of how it is for the Alzheimered brain. My mother is often most confused right after she wakes up. That's when there are imaginary dinner guests coming, some man inviting her out, and so forth. I think she dreams things, but with dementia the line between being awake and being in a dream becomes permeable, and so the dream stays with her and is real while she's awake. We call it a delusion.

And I suspect that as the disease progresses, the already flimsy barrier between the dream world and the waking world tatters and disintegrates like old lace, until it's gone entirely.

Having her home after a nearly six-week absence, after a little taste of having our lives back, is almost worse than if she'd never gone away at all. This is complicated by my refreshed anguish: There's no question that what she's been through has damaged her. I can see that plainly now. It's not just the disease progressing. Though she remembers none of it, the drugs, trauma and abandonment have left her scarred and battered. She's wetting her pants occasionally now. The Depends era has begun, and it's my job to supervise.

I'm not good at this. It embarrasses me, makes me squeamish and miserable. Luckily, she's not embarrassed in the least, nor does she resist. Being a novice to the wonderful world of adult diapers, I go to the store and get the wrong kind—the kind that have to be assembled.

These are for use by people who have lost control of their bladders but who still have their marbles. People who don't have all their marbles will not be able to put the diapers together right, and even if they could, they would forget to wear them. What this means, of course, is that someone else has to do it for them.

No way am I going to diaper my mother. We all have our limits, and this, I'm afraid, is mine. So I devise a way around it: I preassemble the diapers, using myself as a dressmaker's dummy the first time, fitting them over my clothes so I'll know exactly where to put the tabs from then on. Now I can put them together without them having to be on her. The diapers become just like underpants she can step into. I make a couple of pairs every night—one for her to wear to bed, a fresh one for the morning. I lay out the morning pair next to a big note: MOM! PUT THESE ON! THROW AWAY THE ONES YOU WORE LAST NIGHT! And I have to take away all of her regular underpants so there'll be no confusion. It works pretty well. But it's sad, sad, so sad.

And she's waking up really early now—too early for me to get up and cook her breakfast without wrecking myself for the rest of the day. The shortest route to full-blown psychosis for both Mitch and me is lack of sleep, and we're hanging by a thread as it is.

Allen, bless him, is a natural early riser, and available again. We arrange for him to show up at 7:30 every morning (my brother paying him weekly), cook her breakfast, keep her company, take her for a ride, keep her away from the house until 10:30 or so. He never, ever lets us down. Sometimes I hear his car pulling in at the ungodly hour, sometimes I sleep through it. Without him, this stretch of time after her return might have finished us off. Knowing that he will appear, without fail and on time, and that he alone aside from Mitch and me still has some mysterious ability to handle my mother, allows both of us to roll over and steal the two more hours of sleep that probably saved our lives.

"If Someone You Love Has Alzheimer's," says the big expensive ad in the Santa Rosa paper, "Primrose Can Help." I've been looking at this ad out of the corner of my eye for over a year. Santa Rosa, two hours away, had seemed too far. Now it seems just right. The place is not skilled nursing, so her insurance won't cover it, but we call anyway.

Their price is a Steve Forbesian flat rate, the same for everyone—$125 a day. That's just about midway between the cost of the Hostel and the cost of The Pines. It's about a hundred and a quarter short of four Gs a month. So Primrose is pricey, but it beckons. We go.

It's damned nice. It's gated, but subtly so. They manage to make it look as if the gate is there to keep intruders out rather than the inhabitants in. Nice touch.

Alzheimer's is their business. The floors are carpeted, the halls are continuous (if you keep walking, you'll wind up back where you started), there's a central courtyard (read: "corral"). The difference between this place and a nursing home is this: A nursing home reminds you of a hospital. This place reminds you of a hotel. In some ways they're very alike. In other ways they are very different. What are the similarities? Both have halls. Both have rooms off of halls. Both have a lot of people from all over the place converging by circumstance in the rooms and in the halls. Both are institutions. What makes a hotel not a hospital is the absence of linoleum, absence of fluorescent lighting, absence of uniformed medical personnel, and most importantly, the feeling that you are well and are there voluntarily. That feeling is achieved at Primrose by the hotel-like atmosphere. A neat trick, especially when you consider that in an Alzheimer's facility, you are neither well nor are you there voluntarily.

With one flabbergasting exception to the latter. After we've taken the tour, after we've seen the nice shared rooms and the "memory boxes" outside of each room—the clear plastic reliquaries displaying artifacts from a person's intact life, some of the boxes amounting to exquisite little works of art—we sit and chat with Lisa, who has shown us around.

She tells us about a man in residence at Primrose who was a neurologist. He diagnosed himself with Alzheimer's. He put his affairs in order, set up a trust and checked himself in. Mitch and I are both stunned.

Primrose is a fine place. They have a cat who lives in the office and roams the halls. The sordid pissy tragic aspect is way, way less than at The Pines or the place in Davis. Like Dunwood, it's noisy and pleasantly crowded. I'm beginning to understand that what she needs, our only hope, is a big noisy place. I'd send my mother here in a minute. It's the usual problem, though. There's a waiting list. They'll put her on it. When her name comes up they'll meet her, do an evaluation, see if she's a "candidate for their community," necessary because we were forthcoming with them about how she got kicked out of the Hostel and all the rest of it. They'll call. They promise. Don't despair; we know what you're going through, says Lisa. We understand.

The gates clang shut behind us.

Mike, I ask the image now occupying its own extensive memory-box inside my head, what the hell do we do now?

The thing is, Mike could have told me. Of all the people I've known in my life, *he* could have told me. He was so damned smart, so good at weighing realities and options and making decisions. Christ. My mother isn't the only one who misses him . . .

I have a journal of Mike's where he wrote down and developed ideas with an eye to integrating them into various writing projects. The first entry is dated December 10, 1979, just about a full ten years before his death. The last entry, dated November 11, 1989, the night before he went into radical thoracic surgery in San Diego, is a letter to my mother in case he didn't survive. The journal is an extraordinary document. What start out as abstract reflections on life, death, and humankind's place in the biosphere and the universe become intensely personal and urgent as his illness comes on and he finds himself on a collision course with the table, the knife and the heart-lung machine. His own looming mortality brought certain postulations he'd recorded years before into sharp focus and put him to the ultimate test. They say there are no atheists in the foxholes. Well, they're wrong. Mike was in a bad, bad foxhole, but he never showed the smallest inclination to seek refuge in religion or to backpedal from his own clear-eyed sense of proportion pertaining to the importance of a single human life—in this case, his own.

Mike was known as an environmental writer. He was that, but when it came to the popular conception of what "environmentalism" meant, he was something of a heretic. Reading his journal, I find details of what I already generally knew. He asked the hard questions, penetrated into uncomfortable territory where he challenged rampant vague fuzzy

notions, identified myopic self-interest within the movement, and strove
to get a grip on the trickiest question of all—what are human beings,
really, and what's their place in the grand scheme?

A heretic, you ask? He once told me about a theory of his, and how
it shocked people when he put it forth to them, fellow environmentalists
in particular. It didn't shock me. It matched up just about perfectly with
what I suspected from earliest childhood, from the moment I stood there
at the age of four looking down into that grave. What Mike said was that
he believed the reason human beings trash the environment, treat nature
with contempt, is because they see life as a dirty trick. That ultimately
nature is going to trash *them,* so what the hell do they owe nature? I told
him I thought that made perfect sense. He said a lot of people—intelligent, thoughtful people—found the idea too disturbing to even consider,
fellow naturalists and environmentalists especially. Such folk in particular
yearn for order, harmony, meaning. Mike had optimism, cheer, hope—the
qualities of a man who believed in order, harmony and meaning. But he
was willing to face the possibility that ultimately there is none, at least
none that corresponds to our human desires.

And despite the fact—more likely, knowing Mike, because of it—
that nature had played a particular dirty trick on him, dealt him a wild
card in the form of his defective arm, Mike didn't feel vindictive toward
nature. Quite the contrary.

Two major works were taking shape in the pages of Mike's journal.
One he conceived early on: *The View from This Side of the Line* (or, as he
referred to it most of the time, *T.V.F.T.S.O.T.L*). By the "Line" he meant
the line of life and death, the final "deadline." The title is a reference to
a couple of books he'd already put out: *The View from Hawk Mountain*
and *The View from Great Gull.* These were "nature" books, both pertaining to bird migration and populations and laced with Mike's philosophical observations and searching questions.

Mike was known by his pals and colleagues as a passionate "birder."
He'd been impressed by the way my mother whistled while she typed,
and she was impressed by his perfect imitation of the call of the great
horned owl. The two of them spent a lot of time in the woods on weekends out of New York when they were courting. On one of these early

junkets, they'd gone out after dark into the forest to a place near the river that would be a likely owl habitat. They sat quietly, the way you would in a duck blind. Then Mike did his owl call a few times: *Hoo-hoo-hoo-HOO! Hoo-hoo-hoo-HOO-hoo!* (*Who cooks for* you? *Who cooks for* you *all?*) No answer. He did it again. Then someone answered—*ga-LUNK!* A bullfrog on the riverbank. My mother was helpless with laughter, and so was Mike. They sat there in the dark woods, snorting, giggling and gasping until the tears ran.

For most of us, the word "birdwatcher" conjures images of effete twits and little old ladies, silly people in tennis shoes peering through binoculars looking for a yellow-bellied sapsucker or a frog pippit. For Mike, it was pleasure and also serious business. The health of bird populations is a good measure of the health of the environment.

Mike and his birding buddies sometimes got up at 4:00 A.M. and set out on all-day expeditions in all kinds of weather. When there were daytime expeditions that didn't involve getting up at some unthinkable hour, my mother went along, and loved it. They'd count migrating hawks or eagles on a mountaintop. They'd catch birds in nets, "band" them, then let them go so that their travels could be tracked. They'd note down their findings and keep meticulous records. It was jolly good fun and camaraderie, too, of course, a lot like the "bonding" of a hunting expedition, but nothing got killed. It was all in the name of life. Then it would be home, that wonderful satisfying weariness you get from a long day in the outdoors, drinks and dinner and roars of laughter, my mother in their midst, and maybe Mike would get out his guitar . . .

In both of the *View* books, Mike explores the vital link between wildlife research and the survival of humankind in its modern crisis. Such research not only gives us invaluable data with which to measure damage and progress, he felt, but is also a way for humans to develop an utterly necessary *new* spiritual relationship to the planet—one that went, as he put it, "beyond God." You could say that Mike was a deeply spiritual atheist. With *T.V.F.T.S.O.T.L.*, Mike was planning a fairly bold step. He was going to "come out" as a full-fledged philosopher.

The other major work that takes shape in his journal, and which he got very serious about in the two or three years before his death, accumulating a mountain of research and notes, was the Mississippi River book. The core idea was that the great river, flowing the length of the country as it does with countless tributaries, is a virtual alimentary canal of the continent. The condition of the river would be a reflection of the condition of North America after a couple of centuries of human industrialization. Everything he knew would have been incorporated into this book.

I found something in his journal that resonates in an amazingly precise way with my childhood trip to the planetarium when my father had to carry me out screaming: He tells of being a camp counselor in New Hampshire the summer after his freshman year at Harvard. One clear night he was out looking at the sky when he became "terrifiedly" aware of infinite space. He describes the moment as overwhelming, an epiphany. He said that from then on, looking up at the night sky, or even just imagining it, projected him into infinity with neither "floor, ceiling or walls" to protect or stabilize him. *It literally, physically, made me duck, turn away,"* he wrote.

He had pretty much thrown off the Church by the time he had that experience under a starry New Hampshire sky. The moment put a decisive end for Mike to any lingering remnants of formal Christianity in his heart and mind (except, he wrote, for the music). This "space terror," as he so perfectly put it, stayed with him for the rest of his life. He faced it fully, he said, in 1982, when he wrote a lead article for the *New York Times* magazine on astrophysicist Stephen Hawking. He took the assignment not because he had particular qualifications to write about quarks and black holes and dwarf stars, about which he knew little, but because here was a chance to have extensive contact with a man who dealt every day with questions that were huge, important and frightening to Mike. Mike boned up on physics as best he could in preparation and then he and my mother went to England. When they met Hawking and Mike did the interviews, he got a valuable bonus—Hawking, totally paralyzed and in a motorized wheelchair, faced disability, impending death and infinity with apparent equanimity. Hawking knew "space" better than just about anybody, and it held no terror for him. The meeting took place five years before Mike discovered he had blood clots in his pulmonary arteries, before death was more than an abstract inevitability. I suspect that Hawking, without knowing it, helped Mike in his final days.

As Mike's medical problems mounted, so did his desire to live to write the Mississippi book. He was depending on my mother's participation in the project. It would be a celebration of the new lease on their life together. The plan was for Mike to spend a couple of months recovering from the surgery, and then, by spring, the two of them would head for the Mississippi. Mike and my mother had some of their best adventures on the Mississippi during the Audubon expeditions, on riverboats and barges, living with the crews, getting to know the amazing denizens of the river. There would have been more of those adventures. Their camping gear awaited them in the basement. They would have been on the road again . . .

His journal entries in the couple of months before he went into the hospital took on a searching urgency. His mind was going in every direction—off into infinite space, inside his own stricken body, out again to the needy world and the work he wanted so badly to finish for the sake of the world. And of course he was smack up against the dilemma of knowing he was, at best, only postponing the inevitable, and what difference did a few more nanoseconds of Michael Harwood's life make (an "infinitesimal package of matter," as he put it) in the grand scheme of things, in a finite civilization on a finite planet in an infinite universe? For one thing, he knew those extra nanoseconds would make a big difference to my mother.

These were the things Mike was writing about as his personal D-Day approached. His decision to go ahead with the surgery was based, finally, on a sensible, practical, hard look at the statistical chances for survival and recovery as compared to the statistical chances that his condition would, untreated, lead to stroke, early senility, ignominious decline. In other words, living death. He agonized over how my mother would be affected if he didn't have the surgery and turned into an invalid, and he agonized over how it would be for her if he did go through with it and died. They decided together that he'd go through with it. He wasn't going to do anything without her agreement. There's a name for the particular procedure: *pulmonary thromboendarterectomy,* a couple of words that sound to me now like the approaching hoofbeats of Attila the Hun's army.

My mother bounces back extraordinarily from the drugging and trauma. In between complaining about her stomach and asking why Mike had to die when there are so many bastards in the world who deserve to die, she's trying hard. It's infinitely sad for me to hear echoes of the reasonable, conscious, considerate person she once was trying to struggle through the haze. "It's not fair for me to move in on you and Mitch," she says. "I should find an old folks' home."

A friend who lives in Calistoga tells us about a small, very exclusive residence for old ladies up in the high hills above St. Helena. She says it's for refined, educated types, in a private home.

We get Allen to stay with my mother and we go. It's a two-hour drive to St. Helena, a beautiful place saturated with money, and then we pass through town onto a winding climbing forested road, a vista of gorgeous rolling green hills below. And suddenly, we're there. It's a white house with Spanish roof-tiles and a wrought-iron gate. There are no other houses in sight, no cars passing by, just the valley, the empty road, the sky and utter quiet except for a sprinkler chattering away over a golf-course quality lawn.

We pull into the driveway. Hopelessness floods my veins as if an I.V. valve had opened. It's a little like pulling into the parking lot at The Pines, but for entirely different reasons.

We've called ahead. We're expected. A thin, pleasant guy in his forties answers the door and lets us in. The house is gleaming, immaculate—and silent. The man and his wife and two little children share the house with six old ladies. I have no idea where the wife and children might be at that moment. He takes us into the big tastefully appointed living room. At first I think it's empty, but then something moves ever so slightly in my peripheral vision and as my eyes adjust, I see that there are four women in the room. There's a television going, but the sound is off. No one is speaking. They are snoozing or simply sitting in big overstuffed chairs. One of them reclines on a loveseat, knees up and agilely bent. The average age looks to me to be approximately one hundred and eight.

Mitch walks over to the woman on the loveseat, touches one of her knees lightly. Her eyes focus on him in utter shock. He says hello, asks her how she's doing. "I was asleep," she says, and shuts her eyes again.

The man shows us the rooms. Neat, tidy, beds made, bureaus with flowers and family pictures. There's one private room, the rest are shared. He shows us the room where my mother would go if we brought her here. An old lady is sound asleep on one of the beds (sound familiar?). "This is one feisty little girl," the man says, though she looks anything but feisty as we gaze down at her. She looks translucently ancient, fragile, barely breathing. I can see intricate blue veins through the skin of her face and hands. Her hair is white and thin and fine as a baby's. She is—and I am not exaggerating at all here—easily old enough to be my mother's mother.

We get down to business in the kitchen. The man says he'll try anybody for a month. His fee is amazingly reasonable. Tell me a little something about your mother, he says. Is she ambulatory?

Mitch and I both laugh, a little bitterly. Oh, she's ambulatory, all right, I say. And I think: Yeah. Right. I'm going to tell him all about how she pounded on the walls at the Hostel and screamed and smoked and stalked the halls in her underwear and shouted and cursed and walloped someone at the day care program and got put in restraints in a psych ward. Bringing her here would be like turning a Rottweiler loose at a cat show. This was what I suspected from the moment we pulled into the driveway, and now I know it for a fact: She'd lay waste, utterly. She'd destroy this place. Her shrieks would echo off the lovely hills. I can already hear it.

Mitch and I don't have to speak. We are thinking the same thing. We tell the guy his house is wonderful, thank him for his time, tell him we think my mother might possibly be just a tad too much of a handful, thank him again, and beat it out of there. We drive down the long beautiful winding mountain road away from the old-lady aerie and into town, where we find the fanciest bar we can and go in and get shitfaced among the yuppies.

★ ★ ★

"Oh, El," my mother says one night while I'm putting her to bed. "I'll never forget the night when Mike was sick and I rested my head on his chest and he said: '*No, Lovie. It hurts.*'"

And she cries. And I think: No, she probably won't forget that. She'll forget how to breathe and swallow before she'll forget that.

Mike and my mother flew to San Diego on November 5, 1989. They checked into a motel near the hospital, and Mike began more than a week of tests and preliminary procedures. My mother was with Mike for every test where her presence was permitted. He wrote furiously in his journal every day. It's fascinating to witness Mike's courage, and most of all, his unquenchable curiosity as they put him through echo-sound examinations, nuclear lung scans, angiograms and the like. And his writerly eloquence was in high gear. He describes the view of his own beating heart and its main connections on the echo-sound screen thus:

> *Animated gargoyles . . . the white-on-black shadows of pump-ing parts had mouths that said "wow" in regular rhythm . . . delighted to see that although these beats were grossly similar, in details they were visibly different . . . chaos tiptoeing along . . .*

Mike, always thinking of the greater good, and with my mother's blessing, agreed to a couple of experimental procedures in the course of these tests, letting himself be used as a guinea pig. One involved allow-ing his left ("good") arm to be uncomfortably tourniqueted for ten minutes so that blood protein changes when the flow is blocked could be studied; another involved letting them try out a new Doppler imag-ing technique to determine thickness of artery walls.

Every time he underwent a test, some of them queasily invasive and alarming, catheters threaded into arteries and such or down into his chest, he wrote about it in detail, describing what he heard and saw and felt, what the doctors said, how residents and medical students crowded into the room. It's plain that they were ecstatic to have their hands on such an articulate, intelligent and public-spirited patient with such an array of challenging problems.

Even there, in the hospital, facing a ghastly life-or-death ordeal, Mike was clearheaded and his principles were firmly in place. He was acutely aware of his privileged status—that because of his background, education, connections, access to medical insurance and so forth, he was among a tiny handful of people benefiting from a hugely labor-intensive application of cutting-edge life-saving procedures. He questioned whether this lopsided distribution of resources was justifiable, if this was an ethical way for medicine to be practiced. And he had got into the program through the pulling of various strings, getting himself placed in what was already a tight surgical schedule, and so he worried about whether within the small group of patients of which he was now a part he had thrown his weight around—whether or not he might have "bumped" some less well-connected person to a spot behind him in line, someone whose situation might be made more dangerous by waiting.

I drove to San Diego the weekend before the surgery. Tommy flew in from Colorado and Mike's youngest sister, Daphne, flew down from Vancouver. The plan was to have a fun weekend, and then we'd stay for the surgery on Tuesday. Mike would be spending each night in the hospital over the weekend, but he'd be on liberty during the day on Saturday and Sunday, all medical stuff suspended.

We rendezvoused at the motel. My mother had set up housekeeping in the room. She was already on a first-name basis with the motel managers. I slept on my futon on the floor; my brother and Mike's sister had their own rooms.

We had some fun. We rode out to the desert in my big old Ford LTD (big enough to carry all five of us, including my very tall brother) to do a little birding. We went out for a Mexican dinner. We watched movies on the VCR in the motel room. Daphne remarked much later that what she remembers most is how blessedly "normal" everything was that we did that weekend.

There was only one downer, and that was our trip to the much-vaunted San Diego Zoo. It's supposed to be one of the best in the world, with "natural" habitats and so forth, and indeed it's light-years beyond the dreadful prison-bloc zoos of my childhood, but it was a downer nonetheless. First of all, Mike was tired that day, and had to make the tour mostly in a wheelchair, a shocking sight for me. He'd pretty much concealed the fatigue and shortness of breath that were part of his condition. This was my first real glimpse. And he looked pensive and a little sad. I found out later in the day that having to be in a wheelchair was only part of it.

The zoo was a big disappointment. He could see that in some cases the animals had been thrown together in mismatched groups—tropical birds with Canada geese, for instance—and that the "habitats" were cramped and inadequate. But what really got to him was the hummingbird house. This was a cageless aviary designed so that human visitors walked on gravel paths right through it while the birds flew around free. There were only four hummingbirds left. Mike learned from an outraged female attendant that the reason for this was that the hummers, raised by hand and unafraid of humans, would fly right up to people— a lot of them children—who'd then snatch them out of the air and either kill them or take them outside and release them. Some people, the woman said, brought in fresh blossoms to attract the birds, then whipped the creatures to the ground.

I know what Mike was thinking about. He was thinking about his theory that humans are cruel to nature because nature is cruel to them. The Dirty Trick Heresy. Here was a sadly perfect example. It was not what he needed to see on that particular weekend.

He and my mother found out the names of both the curator of birds and the president of the Board of Trustees of the zoo and Mike wrote down the names in his journal. He was going to do something about it. Later. After the surgery.

HOMES—RESIDENTIAL CARE, reads the heading. This is horrible. Surely I've descended to new depths. I'm flipping through the Yellow Pages, looking for somewhere to put my mother, the same place I'd look if I wanted an oil change, a veterinarian or an air-conditioner. How could it have come to this? It makes me quiver with despair.

The names are an invocation of hypnotically soothing euphemisms rich with suggestions of bucolicism: Orchard Park. Walnut Grove. Clover Valley. Coastal Dunes. Brookside. Lakeview Villa. Edelweiss, Sans

Soucee [sic], Meadow Wood, Silver Birches, Sunflower Gardens, Valleyview. Blossom Hill Farm—breeding and sales. Oops! I've wandered into the next heading. Blossom Hill is a horse farm. Too bad.

Some of them have display ads, complete with pictures of blissful smiling senior citizens, promises of scrumptious home-cooked food, stimulating activities, warm and loving care, cheerful cozy atmosphere, beautiful country settings, peace of mind. One of them is on a lake and mentions boat rides. Another offers a rose garden. A rose garden!

It's all in vain anyway. These are board-and-care assisted living places, not skilled nursing facilities or specialized Alzheimer's places like Primrose. And all of them are far, far away, which means when she flipped out, as she surely would, I'd be driving hundreds of desperate miles. Nope. It's going to have to be a skilled nursing facility. I skip a few pages ahead to the Nursing Home heading.

Things are a little more businesslike in this section. A little less glowing, not quite so effusive. Some of the ads make references to comfortable rooms and recreational programs. One of them even claims to have a home-like setting. But that's about as far as they go with that sort of rubbish. A nursing home is a nursing home. Everyone knows that. I see one ad that says "Specialized Alzheimer's Program." The place is in a town a couple of hours away.

I call. Instant brick wall: Sorry, no room at the inn. But if you'd care to leave your name and number . . .

The voice at the other end of the line echoes as if it's bouncing off metal beds and linoleum. Like the place in Davis. I can just about smell the disinfectant over the phone. My mother in a nursing home? It'll be like the geriatric psych ward. Oh, they'll be able to handle her, all right. With restraints and drugs. We're right back where we were.

I cover my eyes, press them into the sockets until I see stars and comets. No nightmare could ever approach this. This is real. There is no way out, no answer. I am being ground between giant machine parts.

She's been back about two weeks now. All the old scabs are ripped open afresh, wounds made worse by our unrealistic hopes that we'd learned something, that we'd get it right this time. All the old sorrow and pity and frustration are right back in place, all the old responses as the same scratchy broken records are played again, in the same old places—the kitchen, the door to my study, the car. Oh, God. The car rides. And her stomach.

When we sent my mother to the Hostel—indeed, the moment we got her on the waiting list—I had a bad feeling about the thousand different things that would surely go wrong. At the top of my list was the fear that the old stomach monster would rise up and wreck everything. It had turned out for us to be the most insidious aspect of her illness during our year-and-a-half struggle. The sorrow, pity and helpless rage had just about devoured me. How could THEY possibly handle it? She'd drive them nuts. Compounding my anxiety was the belief that I'd got myself into a bit of a tangled web—I didn't tell them about the daily grief, the verbatim complaints, the oceans of Pepto-Bismol and Maalox, the fruitless excursions to gastroenterologists. I played it way, way down, said she had an occasional queasy stomach. I fully expected to be exposed as a liar.

But weirdly enough, the word "stomach" was hardly mentioned the whole time she was there and had nothing at all to do with her eventual expulsion. At first, when we made our daily calls to the staff to see how things were going, I asked, as casually as I could, my own guts churning, if there had been any . . . digestive problems . . . ? Only once or twice did they say she'd asked for something to soothe her stomach.

This was baffling, but a huge, huge relief. It seemed to corroborate Mitch's theory that the problem was mainly psychosomatic. Not fake—we both knew her pain was real. But it seemed as if maybe this was proof, finally, that there really was nothing physically wrong. The workings of the Alzheimered mind are beyond enigmatic. Maybe her distress had been some sort of by-product of her mental breakdown, and maybe the stomach era had passed. Maybe it was over.

Wrong. Within a week of her return from the hospital, the sleeping dragon awakes, with renewed fury. It used to be that her stomach was mostly okay until maybe after lunch. Now it starts up first thing in the morning—before breakfast—and sometimes goes on all the livelong day. She comes into the house, lies down on the window seat and begs me to help her, begs to be taken to the hospital, begs for the phone book so she can look for a doctor. Mitch, skeptical of her theatrics, gnashes his teeth, retreats into angry silence. I can hear him slamming his tools around outside. I leap with every clank.

So not only have I put her through medical and psychological torture that would have done a Spanish Inquisitor proud, but she's in worse pain than ever, and my rage and helplessness are back, in direct proportion to that pain, to my guilt and to my anxiety over inflicting this wretched misery and sorrow on Mitch and my anxiety over the urgency of finding a place for her to live and my anxiety over the knowledge that if and when we find a place I'll have to betray her all over again, and then they'll throw her out anyway and we'll be right back where we started. Not a pretty picture. I am often awake and brooding just before dawn in that nasty post-drinking state after short, bad sleep. On trash-collecting day once a week, I lie there and hear the embarrassingly loud and lengthy cascade of bottles coming from the end of our driveway.

And all day, every day, the litany: her stomach, what doctors has she been to, how she wishes she could die, where's her basket, why did Mike have to die, and the latest, heart-rippingest of them all: It's not fair for me to just move in on you. I feel very badly about it. I should find an old folks' home.

I finally bring myself to look at the copies of the nursing notes from both the Hostel and the psych unit. The ones from the Hostel are particularly chilling. They go all the way back to her first weekend there. I flip through them. This is all stuff I know about, of course, but seeing the notes as they were written brings them nastily, immediately alive. They're in the various handwritings of staff people, hasty scrawls that look like graffiti. It's like reading Stephen King: "Constant attention all morning—HELP!" "Tried to strike Rick. Inappropriate behavior almost all nocturnal shift." "New meds. Not bad. Wandering but no signs of violence." "VERY agitated. Screaming in her room at the top of her lungs." "Found walking down hall toward Clarissa's room with lit cigarette." "Up at night, out of room, making threats." "Very confused. Packing things to move. Very agitated. Screaming: WHERE IS MY DAUGHTER? WHERE IS SHE?"

Someone once asked Salvador Dalí if he took drugs. He replied: "Drugs? Drugs? Dalí *is* a drug."

And so am I. I understand that there is only one drug in the world that can keep my mother calm and centered, and I am that drug.

Someone suggests we get in touch with an outfit called the Redwood Caregiver Resource Center. They might be able to help you find a place for your mother, we're told. I call and have a conversation with a black-accented, shrewdly down-to-earth woman named Deborah who wins my heart instantly when I get to the part about The Pines and their $195-a-day "bed hold."

"Bull*shit*," she says spontaneously, and I love her for it. She tells me that Jenny, one of her associates, will be on the coast in a few days and that she'll come for a home visit. Jenny calls. I like the sound of her voice. Like Deborah, she sounds competent, sympathetic, take-charge. A grownup. We make a date. Eleven in the morning next Tuesday.

On Tuesday morning, I get my mother spruced up—fed, hair washed, clean clothes. I tell her a "nurse" wants to ask her some questions. She's always amenable to that, and her lifelong social instincts still kick in—as long as I'm around, of course.

Jenny arrives. She looks just the way I wanted her to look—sixtyish, solid, no nonsense, no frills. She's warm, friendly, smart. I bring her in, sit her at the table, get her some tea. My mother is out in the cottage. I figure Jenny and Mitch and I will talk a little. We'll fill her in on my mother's history and condition and our dilemma and all that, and then bring my mother in so Jenny can meet her.

But it turns out that Jenny is not here to see my mother, though she certainly wants to meet her. She's here to see me and Mitch. We're so accustomed by now to people we take my mother to or who come to the house—insurance guys, nurses sent by insurance companies, admissions people for geriatric facilities, doctors, receptionists—all wanting to question and evaluate my mother that it never occurred to us that someone would be coming to have a look at *us*.

Redwood Caregivers Resource Center is an advocacy organization for—guess what? Caregivers. That group of poor ragged wild desperate semi-demented souls of which we are now senior members in good standing.

God, what a wonderful surprise. Somebody for *us*. We remember why we love northern California. She shows us a questionnaire: "Caregiving Stress—Symptoms and Causes." The first category is called "The Warning Signs of Stress." It reads: "When you experience an unusual level of stress, certain warning signals will occur. Answering the following questions will increase your awareness of these signs. A 'yes' answer to even some of these questions can indicate stress that has become debilitating."

There's a Yes and a No checkbox next to each question, and there are eleven questions under the Warning Signs category. A few samples: Do you feel a loss of energy or zest for life? Yes. Do you feel out of control, exhibiting uncharacteristic emotions or actions? Yes. Do you lack interest in things that were formerly pleasurable? Yes. Are you becoming increasingly isolated? Are you consuming an increased amount of sleeping pills, medications, alcohol? Do you have difficulty falling asleep at night? Are you awakening too early? Do you have thoughts of suicide? Yes, yes, yes, yes, and yes. Christ, yes.

We answer yes to all eleven.

Jenny is impressed. So are we. There's more to the questionnaire, a category called "The Causes of Stress," but we pretty much skip that. We know bloody well what the causes of stress are. We get down to the business at hand: finding a place for my mother. A place where she'll be cared for in a way that will allow me to sleep at night. Jenny has grasped the situation and all its nuances. She starts writing down names of places to call, says she'll be making calls herself on our behalf. She leaves us her card, a pile of literature, a hotline number. I can tell we've moved to the top of her list. She is, as they say, "there" for us.

You can't know the real meaning of that expression until you've spent time in the hopeless hinterlands of the institutional search in the U.S.A. Almost every American will have to venture here at one time or another, whether it's to find a home for an Alzheimered parent or the right place to get lifesaving treatment or to get detoxed or even a place to board your dog. You may find yourself looking in the Yellow Pages.

Whenever you must place someone, or yourself, in any kind of medical/care/rehabilitational/holding facility, you will find, especially in matters that are truly life-and-death, that here, in the richest country in the world, there are no maps, no plans, no guides (unless it's prison, in which case the choice will be made for you), no one in charge to tell you what's the best thing to do. You will be on your own, the way Mike and my mother were. And it will be a good thing if you are a very lucky person.

A couple of mornings later, early: I'm sleeping remarkably well, out cold, far away in a dream, my heavy-duty wax earplugs in place. I wake to Mitch calling out:

"What is it, Mary?"

Amazingly, I'd missed what woke him up: my mother banging on all the doors down the hall until she got to the bedroom door (which we keep locked), shouting in full-on panic:

"WE DON'T HAVE ANYTHING FOR DINNER!"

It's amazing how fast a person can go from dead sleep to up and across the room. Less than a second, I'd say, if they were timing me with a stopwatch.

I open the door. My mother, fully dressed, hair nicely groomed. Looking absolutely normal, except for her eyes: Fear, confusion.

"Mom, it's 6:30 A.M. We were asleep."

"Oh, God," she says. "I'm so sorry. I thought . . ."

Allen arrives at 7:30. Not early enough these days. Not early enough. I send her out to the cottage, tell her Allen will be arriving shortly to cook her some breakfast.

"Allen?" she says. "Who's Allen?"

"You'll remember him when you see him," I say. She leaves, in full beaten-puppy mode. I get back into bed. You really should have gone out there with her, I tell myself. Within three minutes, we hear the front door slam, cupboards banging.

It's pouring rain now. I get up, put on my bathrobe, get an umbrella, find some shoes, take her out, cook her breakfast. She starts complaining about her stomach. Just as I've finished cooking the food, Allen arrives. I go back to the house, drop a Valium, take a few swigs of beer, sleep another two hours. Mitch and I talk about it later. The panic. Total, as if Hutu tribesmen were coming down the driveway with machetes. I try to see it through her eyes: She woke up really early, got dressed, then lay down and slept some more. Woke again, found herself dressed, thought she was waking up from an afternoon nap and the darkness outside was evening. Looked at the clock. 6:30 P.M.! My God! She goes to the house. It's silent, still, empty. No dinner cooking, no Mitch and Ellie, no nothing. We've gone off somewhere, obviously, and abandoned her.

Abandoned her. Which I'm plotting to do. Again.

CHAPTER FIFTEEN

Cry Me a River

On the Sunday night before Mike was to go back into the hospital for the final day of preparation before the surgery on Tuesday, we had drinks in the motel room. Mike's sister would have to leave on Monday morning to go back to work. But we were all together on that evening of the fun day we'd spent in the desert. The docs had said Mike could have one martini.

I'll never forget that martini. *"Dinky for Mikey,"* my mother said, handing it to him. We laughed. Mike half-reclined on the bed next to my mother, leaning on his left elbow, holding the frosty little glass up with his right hand. The "bad" hand. He and my mother clinked glasses and he took a sip, smacked his lips with deep, deep appreciation. It had been a while.

"Mmmmm," he said. "That tastes *so* good."

The next morning, a man weeping loudly in the hospital hallway right outside the door awakened Mike and his roommate at 5:00 A.M. Mike found out later that the man had just learned that his wife was dead. Mike wrote:

> *The first graying of the day had barely begun. I lay in the hospital bed thinking about the irretrievability of events. For us time's arrow goes in only one direction, and what's done is done, what's lost is lost. Even a moment of joy is quickly out of reach behind us . . .*

That night, he made his final entry in his journal. He began:

> *Dearest Mary—If I don't survive the surgery tomorrow, I want you to know that I wouldn't exchange the last 23+ years in your company for anything . . .*

And he ended:

> *What a life I've had! I love you—*

Jenny, true to her word, calls us with contact names and numbers. One place sounds great—a skilled nursing facility near Calistoga housed in a Swiss chalet–type building. The woman I speak to on the phone says that the people there think they're on permanent vacation. Two problems, though: First, they don't have a vacancy just then. Sigh. Second, it's all women.

My mental image of the kind of place where there's even a chance of things working out is coming into ever-clearer focus: I already know it has to be big and busy—Grand Central Station, action and distraction, but not dismal and squalid like The Pines. It should be within reasonable driving distance. And it should take her long-term care insurance. Four Gs a month out-of-pocket is, we now know, the average cost of a specialized Alzheimer's place—with the notable and inexplicable exception of The Pines—and this would run us through her cash on hand quicker than you can say Enron. As much as I like Primrose, the cost—almost 50 Gs a year—is a major and scary drawback.

And last but scarcely least . . . it should have men in it. I now know this is an essential. And I'm not demanding too much of these imaginary men. My fantasy doesn't exactly require that they be Douglas Fairbanks. All I ask is that there be one or two who can maybe speak and walk and who don't require bibs when they eat.

This is a fairly tall order. Anyone who's had any experience at all with homes for the elderly knows that the population is lopsidedly female. Like about eighty percent. Women live an average of seven years longer than men, which means that the selection of men is already pitifully limited numerically, and so the chances of finding a presentable one among that handful are slim indeed. But I can still fantasize, can't I? We've all heard of nursing home romances. Some of the details might perhaps defy the imagination, but we all know they *do* happen. My mother had been courted by lots of men after Mike died, but she hadn't considered a single one of them a serious contender. Perhaps now her standards have been . . . adjusted.

I'm not even necessarily hoping for a romance. Just some masculine company, which had always had a salutary effect on my mother. Someone to offer his arm.

Men or no men, I give the Swiss chalet place our number. They say they'll contact us. Another place sounds just great until they divulge an astonishing and surreal fact, something somebody might say to you in a dream: They don't do laundry. The families have to come get their Loved Ones' dirty laundry, wash it and dry it and bring it back.

"Mike came off the heart-lung machine like a champ," said the thoracic surgeon. This was the same guy who'd accidentally pulled a pack of Pall Malls out of the pocket of his scrubs when we were all conferring a few days before and he'd been reaching for his notebook. "Oops," he'd said, looking down at his hand, quickly pushing the smokes back into his pocket.

Now we were in one of those little family waiting rooms where you sweat it out for hours and hours. My mother had been the most relaxed and confident of us all: Life would not eject Mike Harwood. It was late Tuesday afternoon. They'd started early that morning. It was done. Mike was alive. The doc was happy. My mother was ecstatic. "We got most of the big ones," he said, referring to the emboli. "Want to see?" He had Polaroids.

We crowded around to look.

They were laid out in a display on a white cloth. Purplish, tortuously tubular, about as big around as a fat cigar, like some exotic root or fungus you might see in a marketplace in Canton.

A few hours later we were allowed into the I.C.U. Anyone who can sustain faith in life after death after seeing the I.C.U., who still believes consciousness can somehow exist independent of the living body, should get the Most Out of Touch with Reality award. Here is where the extent to which our bodies are space suits, impossibly intricate vessels of life in a hostile universe, is made manifest. When the space suit's systems are damaged or compromised, they must be compensated for, immediately and precisely, and the staggeringly complicated life-support equipment of the I.C.U. with its choreographed teams of technicians in vigilant attendance is what is required. And as dazzlingly brilliant in function, complexity and wizardry as that equipment is, it's as crude, primitive and unwieldy as a manure spreader compared to the body's micro-circuited and integrated systems. That's why the room is so packed with machinery, and that's why it takes ten or twelve people to run it. When they say intensive, they mean intensive.

So there was Mike. Semi-conscious under the fluorescent lights, suspended tenderly at the center of the life-sustaining web: Respirator down his throat chuffing and hissing rhythmically, catheter, I.V.s, heart and blood pressure monitors, hoses, clamps, wires, sensors, exquisitely acute machinery beeping, whirring, clicking, graphs and arcane greenish readouts moving by on screens, bad arm elevated on pillows, thick, wide vertical bandage on his chest where they had sawed through his breastbone. Deeply, gravely wounded—but alive. I remember watching his eyes as he tried to focus them, and noticing how blue they were.

I also remember being appalled. I'd never been in an I.C.U. before. This, I decided, is a place to be avoided at all costs.

My mother took it with equanimity. All this equipment looked beautiful to her. She was radiant. The surgery was over. He'd made it. He was still on this side of the line, with her.

The next day, Tom flew back to Colorado and I got in my LTD and drove back to northern California. My mother stayed in San Diego. She'd spend her nights at the motel and her days at the hospital. When Mike was sufficiently recovered, they'd come up north for a visit before they went home . . .

Jenny's vigorous advocacy and support keep us from crossing the line. We aren't alone anymore. She is utterly determined, checks in daily, doesn't know the meaning of discouragement, won't allow us to despair. Because we don't despair, we persevere, and perseverance means we are alert and receptive when luck strikes again.

Mitch makes a call to one of his old connections from the time he worked for the state inspecting nursing homes. The woman he contacts gives him—in a violation of policy which could have got her fired—the name of a brand-new place in Vacaville: Sheffield House.

Vacaville? Why does that name resonate in a faintly ominous way? Because it's the home of a famous medical correctional facility for the criminally insane. You hear about some serial killer or rapist getting "sent to Vacaville." Literally translated, Vacaville means Cow Town.

But Sheffield House is not the correctional medical facility. It's a brand-new assisted living place with a specialized Alzheimer's unit. It's big. It's not a skilled nursing facility; no metal beds, no echoing linoleum—but it has something other assisted living places don't have: twenty-four-hour-a-day medical staff. Which means . . . which means . . . which means her long-term care insurance might have to pay for it. With trembling hands, we make the call.

We speak to Megan, the woman in charge of admissions. They have a vacancy coming up in their Alzheimer's wing. Megan is one of these people who seems to have boundless energy and optimism, where they get it I have no idea, and when we mention my mother's insurance company, to whom she's paid thousands and thousands and thousands in premiums over the years, Megan says (and I quote): "Let me call them. I love to take on the big boys."

Megan is not only full of energy and optimism, she's totally simpatico. She pulls our heartstrings from our chests. We pour out our tragic tale to her. She has transcended her job description; she has become, to us, a tower of strength, a confessor and an angel of mercy. Now we have her *and* Jenny. We want to throw ourselves on her, sobbing. Megan takes the insurance company's phone number, says she'll get right on it.

Primrose calls. They have a vacancy coming up, but first they want to assess my mother. One of their people will be in our neighborhood in a couple of days. May she come visit? Yeah, sure, fine, we say, not mentioning Sheffield House. We know too bitterly well how things can fall through just when you think you have them nailed. We set a date.

Megan calls back. She's triumphant. She says it's about ninety percent certain that the insurance company will pay, but we'll have to jump through various hoops first—fill out forms, provide medical records, letters from doctors. Whatever it takes, we say. Whatever it takes.

This is the second time we've assembled a mountain of paperwork and doctor letters for the insurance company. This time, though, we will be trying to accomplish the opposite of what we assembled papers for the last time. The first time, our efforts had been to convince the insurance company that she was not suffering from dementia. Now we must convince them that she is. The fact that she was judged demented by the nurse they themselves sent when we were trying to get her a new long-term care policy is irrelevant; we must start all over again. And we must reinstate certain words we strove to expunge from her medical records before. Specifically, "Alzheimer's."

The Primrose woman comes to see my mother. The meeting goes wonderfully well. My mother is clean and calm and gracious and does just badly enough on the cognizance quiz to demonstrate that she's a perfect candidate for an Alzheimer's facility. "What a doll," says the Primrose woman as she's leaving. "I'd love to have her come live with us. If it were entirely up to me, I'd take her with me right now."

She says she must report back to her superiors and they'll make a decision. We'll be hearing from them within the week. My mother, as usual, doesn't ask who these people are who come and ask her what year it is, to count backward from a hundred by fives, who is the president and to draw a clockface saying ten of eleven (Could you do that?).

Megan is doing everything she can to accommodate us. The usual procedure, for those who are not in an acute state of crazed desperation ("held hostage," as Megan so eloquently puts it) would be that you and the Loved One would come for a visit. You'd see if you like the place. They'd do an assessment, and so forth. Then, if it was yes, you'd go home, pack up, return to Vacaville and set up the room, go home again, come back with Mom when the time was optimal and slide her in like an egg off a spatula.

But Megan says she's sure that there won't be any problem with the assessment, that what I've told her about my mother sounds fine to her. And there's no "bed hold" bullshit à la The Pines. Instead, Megan says to me over the phone: "Do I have your handshake that you want room thirteen?" "Yes," I say. "Yes. We want it." Yes, yes, yes.

For all of these reasons—because of Megan, because of the distance, because it looks as though the insurance will pay, we will do in one trip what should be done in three. We will pack everything and take my mother to a place we have never laid eyes on.

One small impediment: Room thirteen is not quite available yet. Mrs. Kramer, the current occupant, is being evicted because she's become too much for them to handle, but they don't have a place to put her yet, and they are not going to simply throw her out in the street. It shouldn't be more than a few days, says Megan. Monday, probably. This is Thursday. This is a lot like being on a waiting list for a liver transplant: You know that your only chance at salvation depends on someone else's hideous misfortune. I just about fracture my skull on the ceiling every time the phone rings.

Vacaville. I look anxiously at the map. It's hours away, somewhere down between Vallejo and Sacramento. California is huge. My dread and guilt at the prospect of taking my mother up to the Hostel, a ten-minute drive from my house, is nothing compared to what I suffer now. Moving her to the Hostel was a mere practice run by comparison.

I am drenched in anticipatory stress. The rooms at Sheffield House are not furnished, which means we will have to rent a van and drive down there with a big load. Subterfuge and advance preparation will be vastly more complicated. She's bound to notice the van, the furniture, the great distance. What do we say? How do we do this? I remember her pleading calls from the Hostel, her cries of abandonment. And of course, all the recent insults to her person and soul: the drugs, the hospital, the restraints. She feels safe again, and now we're going to trick her and drive her somewhere hours away and dump her. I am torn every way it's possible to be torn. I wish I could tell her she *is* safe, put my arms around her and tell her she's home now, home at last.

And I wish I could get rid of her this instant.

Sunday: Mitch is at the end. He has taken as much as he can. Now, today. This is it. This morning he was in a pretty good mood. But something happened when I wasn't looking. I come out of the bathroom after getting dressed, find him lying on the bed, eyes closed, a deadly quiet dangerous calm emanating from him, a vibe I know too well. At the same moment I hear my mother shuffling across the driveway toward the house. Searching for me, relentless as the Terminator. I leap into my Human Shield mode. This is all my fault. I've brought this into Mitch's life, and I must take it out, immediately, today, this minute.

And I can't. Tomorrow was supposed to be the day. But Sheffield House called on Friday, said Monday was off, that there'd be another delay. They don't know how long. They haven't found a place for Mrs. Kramer yet. She's not just demented, says Megan. The poor thing's psychotic with terror. We've had to call in the State to help make arrangements to place her. This gives me an unhappy little wave of prescience. I can easily imagine the "poor thing" in question being Mrs. Harwood instead of Mrs. Kramer. The tension is ratcheted up another unbearable notch.

I wait by the phone. Primrose calls. They say they'll take my mother on a "trial" basis for a month. I tell this to Mitch; it only jacks up his disgust. A specialized Alzheimer's place and they'll only take her on a trial basis? Fuck them, he says, and lies on the bed staring at the ceiling. My mother comes in and asks about stomach medicines, doctors. I am close to panic. Fifteen mg. Valium and a slug of wine, on a mostly empty stomach, unplugs my terror for the moment.

I know, I just know, it's all going to fall through. And then what? The understanding of things I've only dabbled in before deepens. I'm experiencing some of the interesting processes of mental illness. A small example: I see a truck parked in the neighbor's driveway. As I pass, the words painted on the side of the truck read: PATHOLOGY SERVICES. I look again: It's not "Pathology." It's "Technology." My mind, all on its own, supplied the sinister word.

A corpse swings from another neighbor's porch. Whoops—it's a surfer's wetsuit hanging up to dry.

There have been reports of a mountain lion in the woods around our neighborhood. The woman next door says she saw tracks in the wet ground of the trail behind our house. That trail is where I run. Alone out there, my head filled with loud rock 'n' roll coming through my headphones, I turn around from time to time. The landscape is sun and shadow, trail and woods, perfect context for the sleek tawny green-eyed shape I know I'll see closing the distance behind me. I'm always surprised to find nothing there. I run on, heart pounding, running now like prey before the hunter, expecting at any moment the impact of the heavy body, claws in the flesh of my back and shoulders, fangs piercing my skull. I turn around again: nothing.

I understand that I'm inflicting daily physical and mental damage on myself which could eventually land me in the same condition as my mother, but I'm perversely going ahead and doing it anyway. Talk about stress—now, there's a word I once tossed around casually without the remotest grasp of its true meaning. My wires and fuses are fried, like someone hit by lightning three or four times. I understand that things do not always "work out." People go crazy, commit suicide or mayhem, have heart attacks, breakdowns. It happens all the time. Disaster is an everyday occurrence. Perhaps it is happening to us. Why not? Why should we be any exception? I have lost the feeling I had all my life that I was exempt. Correction: I've almost lost it. Still retain a shred. Still retain a hazy picture of us laughing, happy, prosperous, free. But it's fading. I also know now the extent to which I depended on my mother. In her way, she seemed invincible. That's all over now, obviously, and so certain things in me are collapsing as well. The domino effect. And my prospects look like absolute zero. I feel like a middle-aged failure, looking to myself in the mirror like an Ivan Albright painting.

And Mitch. Ten years older than I, his hopes dashed, saddled with a senile woman not related to him. Oh, how I wanted to set him free. Look at what's happened instead. I'm sure in his deepest, most private thoughts he pictures himself on a sailboat down in the islands, far away from me, my mother and cold rainy northern California.

There's a phenomenon often mentioned in connection with Alzheimer's. It's called "sundowning." It's typical. They get noticeably dottier toward the end of the day. I see it often in my mother. It's the reverse for me: Early morning is when my mental fabric feels as if it's coming apart, and then as the day progresses it knits itself up again. Morning, a magic time for so many people, is the time for me when reality is at its starkest. I'm talking about first consciousness, right when

I pop out of a dream and open my eyes. I can go to bed the night before relaxed and even fairly sanguine, but it's gone by morning.

Illusions are stripped away, and the dilemma of being a mortal being in a vast dangerous godless universe presents itself to me in the plainest way. The waking world seems grim and weighted down with immutable laws of physics and time in comparison to the dream world.

My dream world used to be a great escape, a regular Bijou of the Brain. For a long time I kept detailed journals of my nocturnal Fellini-Castaneda adventures, free gifts, opulent works of art welling up out of my subconscious with the ease and regularity of bonbons from a candy factory. I still dream, but it's a little different now: If I'm not awake in the real world with its leaden realities then I'm slipping, sliding and sinking in some murky, dreary little sepia-toned dream, not even a real nightmare, always at dawn, when I wake as rudely as if someone grabbed me by the hair, full of dread and nameless urgency. Permanent? I surely hope not. One morning I wake to a loud Orwellian voice speaking my name in my head.

During the wait for the call from Sheffield House, the dreams intensify. I catch one of the more interesting ones and write it down. The human brain is a fiction-spinning machine, and it does some of its strangest work at night, in the basement of the mind:

I'm alone, tramping through bleak, bare woods, scrubby trees all around, a cold, raw late-November East Coast feel to the scene. I see tattered remnants of the yellow tape the police put around crime scenes. The tape is shredded, faded and flapping in the wind; whatever happened here was a while ago, forgotten now. No one's around, and no one's going to stop me from going in. There's a big fallen tree lying across a pond. I walk out on it so that I can see what's under the water. I look down below the surface and see what look like big pale bloodless slabs of human flesh and a lot of rubber gloves floating around near the bottom of the pond. Left behind by the medics, I think to myself, and look closer. The gloves are pale and dead-looking like the flesh, with a texture and color like tissue specimens preserved in formaldehyde. They're bigger than normal, and long, too, elbow-length like ladies' opera gloves. Then I notice that in addition to the standard five fingers, the gloves have a little extra appurtenance partway up the wrist, as if whoever wore them had dewclaws like a dog or a cat. Now, that's sinister, I think. Just as I'm pondering this, the tree I'm standing on starts to sink into the water. My tall rubber boots fill and down I go. I start dog-paddling. I know if I don't keep moving I'll absolutely sink. Momentum is the only thing that will save me. I start to swim away from the submerged tree and the gloves, heading toward shore, when I see the dark head of another swimmer in the distance, coming toward me. I must keep moving, or I'll go down, but I also know that if I don't appear utterly carefree and nonchalant, this other swimmer could be dangerous. This is the ultimate acting challenge: It's wintry, the water is freezing cold and I'm in my heavy clothes, but I have to make it look as if I'm just out for a casual swim. Anything else will telegraph "prey" vibrations directly to the swimmer, tripping the "predator" switch inside the brain in the head I see moving through the water toward me.

Getting up, getting coffee, getting to work has always been the antidote. It's been a tendency all my life to brood at dawn, but the year and a half of living with my mother's Alzheimer's has brought it to full fruition. Getting up, getting coffee, getting to work are still the antidote. Not that I'm then a Vesuvius of enthusiasm and cheer, but the mix of brain chemicals that allows me the illusion that things will "work out" is somewhat restored. It's fragile, though, and nowadays it takes very little to plunge me back into a dawn-like despair in the full light of day.

For instance, when my mother asks me, on the same day as the latest call from Sheffield House, why Mike had to die when there are so many bastards in the world who deserve to die.

I've had only two genuine psychic moments in my life. One was years ago when a no-good boyfriend of mine was cheating on me. I saw him and the woman he did it with in a dream. The next day, I mentioned the dream to him casually; the look on his face was priceless.

The other moment was eleven days after Mike's surgery. I was sitting on the bed in my little writing studio looking at the gray ocean and sky and feeling really horrible. Not physically horrible. Horrible in my head. Uneasy, desolate. I'd been having daily conversations with my mother, including one the night before. For the first time I heard something other than optimism in her voice when she gave me a progress report. They were having a hard time getting Mike off the respirator. They'd tried once, but put it back in almost immediately because he still couldn't breathe on his own. You can't speak with a respirator down your throat, so Mike was writing notes, she told me.

Sitting there on my bed feeling horrible, I heard my mother's voice in my mind, a lot like the way you could sometimes hear a faint pre-echo of sound when you put the phonograph needle down on an old-fashioned vinyl record. The phone rang. It was my mother.

"Oh, Ellie," she said. "Michael died this morning."

Died! The word went in like a bullet.

She'd been there to see him. He'd had something he wanted to say to her, but couldn't because of the respirator. She'd stayed with him for a long time, then left the I.C.U. to get something to eat, telling him she'd be right back. When she was returning and was out in the hall, she heard alarms, saw people running toward the I.C.U. She said she knew, she just knew, that it was Mike.

They did everything. Swarmed all over him, opened up his chest, held his heart in their hands, tried to shock and massage it into beating. But new emboli were forming, multiplying, racing though his body—despite the fact that he was so pumped full of anticoagulants that he should have been a virtual hemophiliac.

When they came out and told her he was gone, they asked if she wanted to see him. She said no, God, no, no, I don't want to *see* him! Please, please, just let me out of here. And she fled.

Within hours I was back in the LTD, roaring down I-5, California's main artery. My brother was on a plane. He got there way before I did. He'd already tended to grim business, autopsy consent and cremation and such, by the time I arrived after crawling through hours of heavy snarled L.A. traffic on the last leg. He'd even made the airline refund Mike's return fare. We grabbed my mother, put her in the car and got her the hell out of the motel, out of San Diego and up north to my town.

I'd led an amazingly tragedy-free life up until then. This was my initiation. I remember watching my mother's dazed expression as she tried to process the reality of Mike's death. I saw her come out of a gas station rest room somewhere along the way, looking fairly normal for a few moments and then visibly doubling over, as if she'd been hit in the stomach, as she remembered that Mike was gone, really gone. Mike's suitcase full of his clothes was in the trunk. My mother couldn't bear to look at them, so I put them in the freebox the night we got home.

She stayed with me for a couple of weeks. Then she went to Colorado with my brother, stayed there for Christmas. After Christmas, I got on the train for Colorado where my mother embarked for the long trip to the East Coast. Why did we take the train? One reason was my morbid fear of flying. Another was that my mother wanted to delay going back to Connecticut as long as she could. We thought the train would be a relaxing way to go. I was an Amtrak veteran with at least a hundred missions under my belt, but of course I'd never traveled with my newly widowed mother. It was the holiday season, and the train was packed. We couldn't finagle sleeping accommodations, so we were in seats the whole way. We barely slept. My mother's grief and bitterness tangled around her fatigue as we got closer to home. Her anger was popping out all over and it was getting hard to handle on the crowded train. I had to apologize to the man running the snack bar after my mother flung a tea bag at him because the water wasn't hot enough; I whispered to him that her husband had just died and begged his understanding.

We were supposed to arrive in New York around 8 P.M. or so on New Year's Eve. For some unknown reason we sat stalled in the station in Philadelphia for at least five hours. It was pure Samuel Beckett. Or the premise for a very bad movie. Midnight rolled around and still we remained—bleary, dazed, a few ragged snores here and there. By then there were maybe ten of us left in the car. Someone had a bottle of Scotch. We passed around those little conical paper cups from the dispenser in the rest room, mixed the warm Scotch with a splash of train-flavored water and raised a toast to the New Year, 1990.

It was 1 or 2 A.M. when we got to Penn Station in New York. The city had been having record frigid temperatures, and the cops were letting hundreds of homeless people sleep in the corridors, bedded down along the walls in sleeping bags and cardboard boxes while partygoers in tuxedos, minks and funny hats, carrying noisemakers and half-empty champagne bottles, stepped over them on the way to catch trains to the suburbs. I can't imagine what my mother and I looked like, but it couldn't have been too good, because the party people veered around us deftly, their eyes sliding over us as if we didn't exist.

I would have been happy to lie down on the filthy floor with the sleeping folk, so profound was my exhaustion, but we took a cab to the Yale Club where a friend had arranged for us to spend the night. We had breakfast in the irrelevantly elegant dining room in the morning, then went to Grand Central, got on another train, and headed for Connecticut.

Mike's best friend—the same guy who would accompany my mother on the airplane to California nine years later—picked us up at the station and drove us home. It was a seriously sad and dreadful moment, pulling into the driveway. The big gray house, which my mother and Mike had walked out of almost two months before, waited.

Oh, Ellie, my mother said, hanging back. *I hate this. God, I hate this.*

2:30 P.M., Wednesday: The call comes from Sheffield House. We're clear for tomorrow. The desperate scurrying begins. It's the usual turmoil of emotions: Part of me had been secretly relieved when Megan had called to say there'd be a delay. A reprieve from the governor. I call the car rental place and reserve a van. Mitch and I lay out plans. He'll take her out for a good two solid hours on Thursday morning.

Thursday: I swing into action again, the way I did for the Hostel, but now I must also pack furniture. Table, chair, bureau, pictures from the walls. Again: No Mike pictures. Not even the little one she carried in her wallet. I'm an old hand at this now. Feel a little tougher emotionally. Of course, that could have something to do with the 20 mg. of Valium I popped and washed down with wine. I move efficiently. Brain operating well. Plan the arrangement of the furniture in the space in the back of the van: bureau in first, clothes packed in drawers. Then TV. Then her long table-top placed diagonally, holding TV and bureau snugly in place. Clothes from closet, on hangers, on top of all that. Laundry hamper with big supply of Depends inside, towels, box of books (her novels and her Webster's, especially) basket of toiletries, all tucked into spaces in front of the tabletop. Floor lamp laid gently across the top of heap, all breakable bendable parts supported. Try to arrange and pad for minimum rattling and shifting during ride. Cover everything with old blue U-Haul blanket. Done.

A final but vital touch: I arrange dummy table in cottage so gaping space won't be evident in case my mother goes in there. Two giant old speakers with hunk of plywood across them. Then go inside and lug our extra TV, set it on rigged table at same angle hers was, just the way I did three months ago. Vase of flowers on top, just as it was.

Inside, a fresh whiskey-and-water for me. Fill flask with whiskey for trip, pack lunch into box. Briefcase full of papers, including copy of my Durable Power-of-Attorney. I hear the Toyota's broken muffler in the distance. Mitch and my mother returning. Timing perfect. Here we go.

"C'mon, Mom, let's have ourselves a picnic." That's the part that kills me. It's so easy to get her to go somewhere. She's always ready, eager. Never mind that she and Mitch just got back from two hours of being out—taking pictures, searching fifteen stores, he tells me later, for a new basket for her—all I have to do is say "picnic," and she's ready. She trusts me completely.

"Let's not forget my folding chair," she says.

Just as I anticipated, she does not notice the stuff covered with the blue U-Haul blanket in the big space behind her seat. Nor does she ask about the shiny brand-new van.

It's a gorgeous day. Wall-to-wall blue.

"Eleven fifty-six," says Mitch as we pull out of the driveway.

It's a gradual deception, its success depending utterly and insidiously on her zero short-term memory. Our story evolves as the trip gets longer and we get farther from home. Instead of stopping for our "picnic," I pass out sandwiches in the car. She's complaining a little about her stomach, but the food and the fantastic scenery of Rt. 128 through the Anderson Valley (the hills of heaven, if they existed, could not be more beautiful than this part of California) divert her. Mozart on the tape player. My discreet little cup of whiskey-and-water on the floor. The only way I can do this. The only way.

Our story changes as her questions change.

"Where are we going?"

"I've been working hard all week, Mary," says Mitch. "I wanted to get out. Have a change of scenery." She accepts this. Doesn't ask about the picnic. We drive on. Talk about the gorgeous trees, hills, sky. One hour. Two. Soon we're through the idyllic Anderson Valley and onto the freeway. Things looking a little more businesslike. Keep that Mozart playing. Oh, Wolfgang, I think; is there any way you could have known how your music would serve in the two centuries after your short, short life, how it would save people's sanity, and more—literally get them through life-and-death predicaments?

"Where are we going that's taking us so far from home?"

"We have some business to conduct down this way. Stuff we've gotta do." This, too, she accepts.

Soon it's time to start consulting the map. Follow the signs for Vallejo, then Vacaville. We're making good time. I'd expected it to be a much longer trip. Mitch and I mutter to each other about signs, routes, exits. I'm relieved to find Vacaville not quite the flat ugly nowheresville I'd pictured. Rt. 80 carrying us there goes through some rather lovely craggy hills.

"Tell me again where we're going."

"Well, Mom, you know how your stomach's always bothering you and you feel dizzy and off-balance sometimes?"

"Yes?"

"Well, we're going to take you somewhere where they can look after you and where it's close to a good hospital so we can get to the bottom of the problem."

This is not a complete lie. Her stay at the psych unit in Petaluma may have produced one useful piece of information: A test they did indicated a possible water-on-the-brain condition. Further tests are necessary to confirm the extent of it. One nurse there, whom we liked and who seemed to be the only one there with anything on the ball, said there could definitely be a connection between the hydrocephalus and her increased urinary incontinence. Other things, too, maybe. By serendipitous coincidence, I heard that my old school roommate's husband had water on the brain last year, his case severe and much faster, but all kinds of symptoms similar to my mother's: memory loss, nausea, vertigo. He had surgery, a shunt put in his head.

We've talked about it: Do we pursue this? How? When? Brain surgery, a shunt in my mother's head? Do we put her through that or do we just let it go because she's old and has dementia and we're burnt out? But what if this is the cause of most of her problems? What if this is why she has a queasy stomach all the time, and is peeing in her pants more frequently? Her doctor did not seem to think there was any great urgency, unlike the nurse at Petaluma. Said he'd let us know when the "team" that tests for this sort of thing comes up our way. Down here, there would be no waiting for such a traveling show. Vacaville is near some of the best medical facilities in California. Get her settled, I think to myself, then get her tested for this, maybe treated. What if . . . ?

So that's our story when we pull into the driveway at Sheffield House. The picnic is long, long forgotten. The place is huge and new, adobe stucco and red tile roof. Looks like a nice big hotel. Front desk like a hotel, spacious, gracious lobby.

We meet Megan: Small, dark, pretty. A nurse interviews us. My mother, accustomed to medical questions, oddly acquiescent to our quasi-credible story about why she's here. Lies down on the couch, says she's exhausted. We're served fancy tray of iced tea and cake and fruit. I'm sweaty, grubby, desperate. Answer questions, scrawl my signature here, there and everywhere, stuff cake into my mouth. Mitch has disappeared to unload the van. Conversation with Tommy on phone about money. Put Mom on. She's pathetically glad to hear his voice. Makes me feel a little like chopped liver, but that's the familiar syndrome among caregivers. You, the one in there with your sleeves rolled up doing the dirty work, sometimes feel a little . . . unappreciated.

Mom puts on a pretty good show. I tell the nurse about the drugging at the Hostel and at Petaluma. Urge them to try to resist medicating her. Just get her through the separation anxiety without drugs if you possibly can. Mom asks where the ladies' room is; gets up, follows nurse's directions, finds it, returns to the office, all unassisted.

Then Megan escorts us to Kingswood Court, the in-house Alzheimer's/dementia unit. She tells us my mother will not be entirely segregated from the non-demented residents who occupy the rest of this huge structure. There's a group of them in the lobby; old people with all their marbles, sitting on couches around a glass table, a couple of the women positively elegant.

We go through the lobby, walk down a long hall. Pass a huge dining room with crystal chandeliers. Like a cruise ship, I say.

Kingswood Court is entered through a door where a simple code is punched in whether you're coming or going. Noticeably less grand and distinctly uncourtlike, but nowhere near the level of grimness I've seen in other places. No chandeliers in this dining room, but her room is a fabulously pleasant surprise: a lot like her room at the Hostel minus the balcony, a little bigger even, nice high ceiling, and with a private bathroom! I had expected her to have to share a bathroom, but here, a glorious and fine bathroom with a huge shower, big enough to accommodate a wheelchair. Mitch has arranged all her stuff while I was in the office signing papers. It looks damned fine and cozy. Her table, her dictionary, pictures set up in the bookshelf.

The usual whimpers and protests. This is *my* room? I'll be staying *here?* How long? But soon it's time for dinner. We're invited to eat. The food vastly inferior to the Hostel food, like school cafeteria food, but I'm not complaining. Chicken strips, coleslaw, french fries. We wonder if the people eating under the chandeliers are getting the same food. But Mom seems not to notice or care. We get a look at the inmates: A lot of them are surprisingly together. One strange skinny nerdy dude, with glasses and a distracted look like a physicist with formulae on his mind, youngish compared to the others, who keeps getting up and sitting down. A very old lady in a wheelchair who demands that Mitch come talk to her; tells him that he has to move her from this table to a different one. He demurs, pats her on the shoulder. At another table, some amazingly normal-looking men—not in wheelchairs, not drooling. I've already noticed that Mom's next-door neighbor is a man. There's a picture of him outside his door in his WWII uniform. Don't know which of the guys in the dining room he might be, but it allows me a shred of hope.

She's catching on that we'll be leaving her here. That expression on her face. Her lip quivering.

"But I want to be in a place where I know the people!" That lovely fantasy: a retirement home in Connecticut, a nice Victorian house, on the village green, peopled entirely by her old friends. Wish I could cast a spell and make it so. Of course, if I had that kind of power, I could also bring back Mike and cure her illness . . . and we sure as hell wouldn't be eating french fries in Vacaville, California.

"But Mom," I say feebly. "You can make new friends! You've gotta give people a chance!"

Back to her room. Elena, one of the staff, brings a resident named Donna with her. High-functioning, tiny, wizened, kindly.

"Come on, Mary," says Elena. "Donna will show you around."

My mother looks at us.

"You'll be here when I get back, won't you?"

"Of course," I say, thinking it was true when I said it.

They go. Megan had advised us that cold turkey was the way to do it. Mitch and I watch: The last I see of my mother, Donna is holding one of her hands and Elena the other and they're going down the hall. Dorothy on the yellow brick road. We look at each other, tacitly concur, and flee like thieves for the exit door. Punch in 2-4-6-8 Star and beat it out of Kingswood Court.

In the car, on the freeway, we pass the flask back and forth. Do not judge us, Gentle Reader. You'd have done the same, I promise.

We stop in Cloverdale, the town at the junction of Highway 101 and Rt. 128. We go where we always go when we pass through Cloverdale, the Quikstop, a gas 'n' grub kind of place, teenagers in the parking lot, brilliant fluorescent lights inside, but over the years I've developed a genuine fondness for it. Great restrooms, private, you can lock the door. A real little oasis whether you're headed for home or away from it. Mitch is looking forward to getting a couple of their delicious greasy nitrate-soaked meat by-product hot dogs. I get a tamale. We buy the largest, cheapest bottle of beer we can find in the cooler: Budweiser. The turn in the road that puts you on Rt. 128 always brings a surge to the hearts of people who live in our town on their way home. You can pick up the local public radio station loud and clear. And if you're in the mood, you can drop in at the station, which is right on 128, about halfway home.

Tonight, it's a rock 'n' roll show. The DJ is way in the groove, doing that magic thing that a DJ does when he's really on it: Plays songs as if he's playing them just for you, reading your mind. It's dark, the familiar road with its hills and twists and turns carries us along in the friendliest way in our smooth, gorgeous rental van. We pass the Budweiser back and forth. I love good rock 'n' roll as much as I love Mozart. I have a small epiphany: The past eighteen months have aged me, driven fatigue and ennui deep into my bones, wrung out my brain. What I need, I realize, is rock 'n' roll therapy. I get from good rock what some people get from religion: inspiration, rejuvenation. Hope, even. By the time the DJ gets to the Traveling Wilburys (old masters Bob Dylan, George Harrison, Roy Orbison and Tom Petty got together, fooled around, made one of the great albums of all time) I know it's The Truth.

We get home, drink some more, just because. I prowl around the house for a while. Mitch falls into bed and goes instantly to sleep. I'm intensely aware of the dark empty cottage outside, my mother's stuff strewn around, stray clothes left behind on hangers, shoes she can't wear anymore because they hurt her feet.

Shoes. You feel so goddamned sorry for shoes. They carry a peculiar pathos when they become left-behind objects. I've seen the power of shoes in a couple of exhibits. There's a huge pile of shoes in one of the Holocaust museums, and I remember a vast display of the shoes of gunshot victims as part of a handgun-control rally in Washington, D.C. Tomorrow I'll deal with my mother's shoes. There's plenty right here in the house to jerk the old tear ducts. Here are her bouquets on the shelf over the sink and on a windowsill. Here's a half-finished crossword puzzle, here's her bottle of Pepto-Bismol, a remnant of her daily stomach struggles, possibly the winner of the What Made Ellie, Mitch and Mary Craziest Contest since late October 1998. But the sentimental cripple seems to be getting a little tougher. I can contemplate these potential snares with fair equanimity.

I finally go to bed. I dream: I'm walking along a road in my hometown in Connecticut. Feeling a little bleak; it's some bare, muddy season there. I look down at my feet. I'm wearing my mother's worn-out grubby old blue-flowered bedroom slippers.

CHAPTER SIXTEEN

Sunset, Children . . .

May: I'm on an airplane, flying from San Francisco to Hartford, Connecticut. I'm wedged in tight, at the end of the row, next to the window, which I specifically asked for. I hate flying. A few years ago, I was on one of those wide-body planes with a center section of seats, and I discovered that my misery and terror were about a hundred times worse when I couldn't look out the window. So now I know—it's absolutely necessary for me to have a window seat, even if it means being stuck for the entire flight, which I am: My two seatmates are nuns. Large nuns.

When I saw them coming down the aisle while the plane was loading and I was already in my seat, buckled up and full of Valium, I just knew they were heading right for me. And I was glad. A person in my condition will grasp at anything.

Nuns? Fantastic! The plane can't possibly crash if I'm sitting next to nuns! I might add that I'm wearing a white scarf given to me at a Save Tibet affair a couple of years ago; that, too, is going to keep the plane from crashing.

It so happens that I have a cousin who's a nun. I was aware of my face getting ready to greet the nuns—as they would surely greet me— to chat with them, tell them this little bit of lore. I felt just like my grandmother, who was famous for starting up conversations with people on buses, elevators, street corners. My mother sometimes got impatient with this. You always knew when my grandmother was about to swing into action; you could see her mouth arranging itself, a little preparatory movement of her throat, her eyes drawing a bead on her quarry. Many was the time I saw my mother put a firm hand on my grandmother's arm: "No!" she'd whisper fiercely.

But the nuns just sat right down without a glance in my direction. They settled themselves, snapped on their seat belts, reached into their bags and pulled out Bibles.

Wrong. Danielle Steel novels.

Fine, I thought. Between the white Tibetan scarf, the nuns and Danielle Steel, what could possibly happen? Sitting with nuns is going to make it a little harder for me to swig from my jar of bourbon-and-water Mitch has thoughtfully put in my bag, but I'll manage. One thing I've perfected in recent months is furtiveness, for which I have a natural talent anyway.

I have to sit next to the window when I fly, and I also have to drink. I don't have a choice. Especially when I'm on my way to Connecticut to empty my mother's house. My emotions jumped around like fleas in a frying pan as we taxied. *Here we go*. Next comes the perversely sensual rush of pure distilled fear when the pilot's got the plane positioned for takeoff, and you can just about feel the machine contracting the muscles of its haunches, and the engines rev to their full awesome power and then you're pressed back into your seat with the roar and the speed and there's no turning back . . .

It turns out that the nuns don't give a hoot about my jar; they read their books for the entire four hours and fifty-five minutes without looking up.

My mother had been gone from her house for nineteen months when my brother and I go back. It's been twenty months since he and I had been there last. Even though a lot of the furniture and other stuff had already been sold, and various housesitters had been in residence, I know that her office is still crammed full of her papers and books and Mike's papers and books, their camping gear from the Audubon trip is

still in the basement, her dishes and pots and pans are still in the cupboards and her clothes still hang in the closets. And there will be shoes
. . . lots of shoes.

I'm going into the heart of the beast. That old Connecticut
Melancholia is looking like a black hole now.

At least it isn't autumn. This time, it's the last week of May. The leaves
are fresh, and as green as a katydid's wing, but it's chilly and the skies are
sullen. Tommy's already spent a couple of nights alone in the house when
he picks me up at the airport. I imagine what it's been like for him.
Church bells, crows, wet tires on the road . . .

I can replay other sounds in my head too: the big heavy antique front
door of my mother's house, that made a rattle and a squeal when you
opened it and shook the walls when you slammed it. I can hear the ring
of her old wall-mounted rotary phone, her businesslike and emphatic
whir-clickety-clickety when she made a call, the sound of the screen door
to the back porch, the scrape of the dining-room chairs on the wood-
en floor, the squeaky toilet-paper roller in the second-floor bathroom,
the clunk-gurgle of the toilet flushing.

And my mother's footsteps on the top floor.

Every house has its own smell. And even though smells are the most
powerful memory-evokers, it's oddly impossible to remember a smell
the way you can conjure a sound, a sight or a touch. But the instant a
smell hits your nose you're there. It's time-travel. My mother's house has
a complicated aroma: spice, food, dust, a not unpleasant hint of mildew.
A moist organic back-East aroma, definitely not anything you'd find in
California.

Tommy pulls the big rent-a-car into the driveway. In the past, the
light by the front door would have been on and my mother would have
been standing there, ready to fling her arms around us. Many, many's the
time I've arrived here after traveling a great distance after a long
absence. This has been by far the longest absence, and certainly, figura-
tively, the greatest distance. It's almost always night when I arrive, the
way it is now.

I get out of the car. It's like stepping out of a spaceship in a Ray
Bradbury story, where people land on places like Mars and find eerie re-

creations of their hometowns: Here's the road, the trees, the streetlamp, the Connecticut night air with its moisture, odors and sounds, all untouched by time. And the house, dark and waiting. If this were a Bradbury story, my mother would be there in the door. But she's not. That's how I know it's real.

My brother and I walk into my mother's house. SKREEEK, BAM! goes the front door. I'm feeling ghostly—desolate, displaced, treading the floors of my ancient home. Maybe we *are* ghosts, and don't know it. The house is dark and smells the same as it has for forty years. Tommy flips on a light: Everything has that shrunken, diminished look that places take on when you come back after being gone a long, long time. And of course, half the furniture is missing, hauled away by the auctioneers a year and a half before. The first thing we do is head to the kitchen for a drink. Look at those ghosts: They walk right through the wall as if they don't see you.

I sleep in my mother's room. Tommy has set himself up in the guest room at the other end of the hall. I lie in her bed (minus the antique brass frame), my head buzzing with exhaustion, alcohol, Valium, the residual roar of jet engines and the weirdness of being at the other end of the continent in the space of a day. I listen to the house.

It was built around 1860, and it sighs, creaks, whispers and occasionally thumps and thuds mysteriously. It has an oil-burner in the basement and old-fashioned radiators. On winter nights, the pipes clanked and banged and the radiators hissed and made eerie little high-pitched wails, barely within the range of hearing. When I was a highly suggestible and imaginative child, I'd put my ear close to the radiators and listen to the sound, like the whine of mosquitoes but higher and thinner, and it sounded to me like tiny human voices, transmitted from far, far away, trying to get a message through.

When I was a kid I used to worry a lot about my mother dying. Not that I thought she was going to die imminently. But I knew that some day she would, and I hated that fact. By the time I was seven, I'd learned enough arithmetic to do calculations—I broke years down into months, months into weeks, weeks into days, days into hours, hours into minutes, and presented myself with likely numbers measuring the remaining span of my mother's life. And now here I was. I'd arrived in the distant future, in the next century, three hundred fifty-nine thousand one hundred sixty-one hours later, getting ready for the final dismantling of her life, and mine, and my brother's, in this house.

I sleep long and late that first morning. Wake up in my mother's bedroom, the spring breeze rustling the curtains. I roll over on my back. Tommy is up, cooking breakfast downstairs. Aromas waft. On the wall next to the bed three pictures hang. For forty-three years, there have been three pictures. Two of them have been there for the entire forty-three years; one of them has hung for only twenty-four years, replacing its predecessor. In the center, a big elegant gold-framed photo of my great-grandfather Colonel Alexander Bacon, around age thirty, sometime in the 1880s, I believe, looking splendid in his full-dress uniform, complete with gloves, sword and polished boots, posing against a painted backdrop and a bearskin. That one has always been there. To the left, a picture of my grandmother, his daughter, as a toddler, 1892 or so, her hands in a miniature fur muff. That one has always been there, too. The one on the right is the newcomer—a picture of my grandmother as a lovely young woman with shiny dark hair coiled on top of her head. My mother put that one up and took another one down when Mike entered her life and bedroom. The one she took down was a picture of Tim Durant (who was born in 1900) around age five, holding a toy drum, blonde ringlets cascading, the same wise-ass expression on his face that he'd wear for the next eighty-one years.

I'd seen the box of her erotic journals as recently as three or four years ago. It's the first thing I look for when I get up that morning. I go into the little room next to her bedroom and stick my arm into the dark place around a corner in the back of the closet, where she had hidden it, but it's gone. Removed and destroyed, I'm sure, by her own hand, in the couple of years before she started losing her mind. Too bad. Some of her best work was in that box.

But the closet is far from empty. It's packed with her clothes. For the entire year and a half that she was with me, she talked about her clothes almost every day. If it wasn't nameless women moving them out of the house, then it was a storage facility where she herself had put them. Wherever they were, they were a source of longing and anxiety to her. Not because they were fancy or irreplaceable. They were just everyday clothes, but they occupied a hugely important place in her mind. I have to go back to Connecticut and go through my clothes, she said a thousand times. And who took them out of my house? Once, in a vain effort to lay her chronic anxiety to rest, I'd even called her house-sitter with her right there in front of me and asked him where her clothes were. I moved them all to the ironing-room closet, he'd said. Everything. And here they were—and all her shoes.

This is a weird little room. Cluttered, unheated, neglected, in a far corner of the house on the top floor, the paint on the windowsills peeling, the curtains tattered and water-stained. The door was always kept shut. No one ever spent more than a few minutes in here. You always went in, did what you needed to do, then got out and shut the door behind you. You had to climb over boxes, laundry baskets, the vacuum cleaner, broken lamps and a big pile of blankets and sleeping bags to get to the ironing board or the cupboards holding the sheets and towels.

The cupboards are a piece of history. They were designed by Durant himself to hold his shoes and riding boots. This room had been his "dressing room." He had chosen the curtains and the dark beige paint still on the walls and crumbling from the sills; he had designed the shoe shelves, cupboards and closets with their brass fixtures. I believe that the old Durant vibes had a lot to do with why this room was to be lonely and bereft for the forty years after his departure. It was mildly haunted, certainly unloved. And cold. The radiator never worked in here.

There are other Durant remnants in this room, even now: a few ancient monogrammed towels, monogrammed shoetrees, mono-grammed wooden coat hangers. He'd had monogrammed bathrobes, monogrammed clothes brushes. My mother had always been scathing about the futile vanity of monograms. She once said, What do people need them for? To remind them who they are? But she'd married a man for whom monograms were essential. To remind him who he was, I guess.

Durant's vanity and aspirations to country squiredom could be a big pain on a purely practical level. He considered American cars low-class, and so we drove a series of little English cars (also monogrammed). They may have made him feel like gentry, but they were flimsily built in that era and broke down constantly, stranding us in rural Connecticut and New York State towns trying to find British fuel pumps and such, and on frozen winter mornings their crummy little engines r-r-r-r-r-r-r-r-r-r-ed until the batteries ran down. It's a damned lucky thing we were never in a crash in one of those tin-and-cardboard contraptions. He drove like a crazy man, which of course is what he was.

I leave the room and close the door. One of my jobs will be to go through her clothes. And down the hall, waiting for me like King Tut's tomb, is her study.

Tommy has done a lot of work in the couple of days he's been here by himself. He's got the services of a guy called a "picker." This is quite a deal: *He* actually pays *you* and then he empties out your house. Most of the stuff will go to the dump, and he drives the load there and pays the dump fees. Of course, he's hoping to make a profit by snagging some valuables along with the junk. So before he makes his offer, you haggle. You go through the house together and hammer out an agreement. Along with the good stuff, he has to take the lowliest detritus. That means old tires, cans of dead paint, sprung mattresses, broken furniture. Everything.

My brother's made the deal with the picker. The picker's happy. He's getting most of the books—and there are some really good ones—some very sellable furniture and a selection of choice pieces they've shaken hands on. He'll pay us $500 and empty the place completely. The pieces Tommy's decided to keep he's separated out and organized into an impressive display in the living room: an antique Chinese plate that had belonged to my mother's iceberg of a father, some tall fancy brass candlesticks, some prints, a couple of oil paintings, a fancy little inlaid bureau, some silver, an ornate old accordion Mike gave to my mother one long-ago Christmas but which, mysteriously, she put away and never played. There's a gorgeous tall gold-framed full-length mirror that's hung in the front hall since the Durant days. Antique dealers are going to come look at these things, make offers. Tommy and I have agreed: We'll be mostly ruthless. We will resist sliding down into the sinkhole of sentiment. We will not ship furniture across the country. We will liquidate. The money will go into my mother's account.

A couple of "dealers" show up that first morning. They look like Hell's Angels in civvies. They inspect the array. They don't talk much, except to grunt to each other in some sort of code. They act as if the things on the table are garage-sale rejects. They look at the mirror, say they could get a better one at K-Mart, offer $50. Forget it, says Tommy. They leave.

Another guy shows up later, immediately offers $600 for the mirror and good prices for a few other things. Done, says my brother. Women have always liked their reflections in that mirror, Tommy tells the guy.

And so it goes. We know that my mother had sold some valuable pieces to unscrupulous sorts like the first two in the couple of years before we got her out of there. And sometimes she lost the money. Just plain lost it, right there in the house. I recall a mad scramble on a visit a few years ago, searching for a thousand bucks in cash that she said she'd tucked away but couldn't remember where. She used to hide money in *Murder for Profit,* but not this time. We ransacked every book, every drawer, every pocket, every shoe, but never found it. Knowing what I know now, I understand that we might have been chasing a mirage.

My mother's study will be my province. I'm hungry to find certain things, and this is my last chance. I'm looking for that stash of her writing—those unpublished short stories, her "Yours in the Flag" letters, a never-finished novel—buried (I hope) for decades beneath the geological layers. I haven't seen the stories since I was eleven or so, but I want them all. Bad.

And of course, the original big glossy photo of John Huston kissing her at the wedding.

Since we were last here, André, at our request, had emptied Mike's study, cramming everything of Mike's into my mother's already-packed study on the top floor. Now it's truly formidable. The remnants of their lives and work are all mingled, tangled, jumbled and stacked in this small room. It's a shrine to *kawaisoo.* We could seal this room in Plexiglas and put up a velvet rope and a plaque.

Ah. But it's only the very few of us who get the velvet rope and the plaque, the room left as it was the last time we walked out never to return. The quill and the eyeglasses lying next to the open book, the shawl draped over the chair . . .

Most of the time, it's the heartsick offspring wading in to do the sad, sad duty. Sadder, in its way, because my mother is not dead, but everything we are doing is exactly as if she were. This is Ground Zero, and I'm about to begin excavation. I'm going to have to toughen up fast.

When we had last been here, and Tommy and I tried to start going through the things in her study, and she'd stopped us. She was trying to defend herself, as she would a lot over the next year and a half.

The memory I'll be stuck with forever (or until I get Alzheimer's myself) is of my brother and me chasing my mother around the house while she shrieked and cried that she wouldn't go. Maybe someday they'll perfect laser micro-surgical-specific-memory removal. I'll say, Please expunge the memory of us chasing my mother. And let's see . . . oh, yeah—the memory of my mother in restraints at the geriatric psych ward. And the memory of her standing in the driveway in the rain, shouting, *You don't want me!* And as long as you're in there, could you maybe clean out that memory of the brochure I saw on dog and cat cruelty in restaurants in China? Okay, Miss Cooney, they'll say. Just put your head in the apparatus and hold very still . . .

But she wasn't here now to defend herself. I went in and started. I just picked up a handful and started.

The picker has an assistant, a taciturn fellow named Paulie. The picker, Bobby, talks enough for the both of them. Bobby is friendly and outgoing, asks a zillion questions. Paulie doesn't even make eye contact. He lifts heavy objects and follows Bobby's orders.

They've parked Bobby's big truck in the back yard. They work like stevedores. They fill the truck, load after backbreaking load, take trips to the dump and to Bobby's warehouse. One day around lunchtime Tommy offers them beers and we all go sit out on the deck overlooking the beautiful river valley.

Bobby asks us where our mother is now.

"She's in a home in Vacaville," says my brother.

Paulie perks up, speaks for the first time.

"Vacaville?" he says. "California?"

"Yeah," says my brother. "California."

"I done some time in Vacaville," says Paulie, looking at his hands.

We're pretty sure he doesn't mean Sheffield House. We suspect it's the State Correctional Medical Facility he's talking about. This is a serious place. Charlie Manson spent some time there a while back.

"Uh—what were you there for?" asks my brother. Paulie considers for a moment.

"She shoulda left me alone," he says, still looking at his hands.

Bobby laughs the nervous laugh of someone privy to a secret, and Tommy and I gaze silently at the view.

There's a handsome doorknocker on the front door. It was one of my mother's great finds—brass, a feminine hand gracefully holding a sphere. Tommy has taken it off the door. It's too good to leave there for the new owners, who've nickel-and-dimed us on the house deal to the point where it nearly fell through. There's a hole where the knocker was.

An old guy, Frederick, an antique dealer, has befriended us. He drops by every couple of days to see how we're progressing. He's a kindly fellow, sympathetic, concerned about the amount of work we're doing in a mere ten days, when the new people will take possession. We're kindred. We all grew up in this neck of the woods and remember when dairy farms dotted the landscape and Swamp Yankees ran the local government. He sees that the doorknocker is gone, and shows up on one of his visits with a replacement. Nothing as elegant as the original, just a plain brass ring, but it covers the hole. Little stuff like that can ruin a deal, he says. Now they won't even notice.

Word spreads fast that we're there. Friends of my mother's, some of them people I've known all my life and who knew my mother all the way back to her girlhood, drop by. One woman, just about exactly my mother's age, starts visibly at the sight of me. She looks as if she's going to burst into tears for a moment. Oh, she says, I can't tell you what it's like for me to see you, looking so much like your mother . . .

Another woman, a sturdy tan tennis-playing widow, steps into the front hall without knocking and calls out, just like the old days. I know for a fact that this woman is eighty-one or so, several years older than my mother. Aside from her sun-wrinkled hide and white hair, there's nothing old about her. Her mind is perfectly intact. She's wearing shorts. She's just come from a tennis game.

Her own husband died about fifteen years before. She's thrived in widowhood, the way a lot of women do. They're sad for a while, but then they get over it and a sense of freedom sets in. Sometimes it's downright relief—life is noticeably pleasanter with the old man gone.

Ah. How I wish my mother could have been one of those sturdy tennis-playing widows, one of those women who learns to use a computer, does e-mail, studies a new language, goes on treks to Tibet . . .

Another old friend who stops by is a man my mother's known since she was a teenager coming here for the summer. He was part of the local crowd she ran with back in the late 1930s. Square dances (the caller was a Swamp Yankee named Tude Tangway), rides over the line into New York State where the drinking age was eighteen, midnight dips in the lake. He looks damned good for a man of seventy-eight—flat stomach, broad shoulders, slim waist. Hard physical work can do that for you. I know something about this guy. He's married, has been forever, but sometime in the 1960s or so, he was dancing with my mother at a party and he whispered in her ear, *"I've always loved you, Mary."*

He invites us to come have dinner with him and his wife. We've known her all our lives, too. We have a lot of dinner invitations now. People are fantastically attentive. And as this, our old home, gradually empties, our lifelong second home, the Chernov house, is where we go just about every day. Alexis and Katrina are long gone, and André is the master of the house, but they're both entirely present in him. He has her mad blue eyes—except that he's not mad at all—and he has his father's large strong veiny Michelangelo-designed hands and arms.

Walking through the door there is to step through time. In the midst of this world upheaval, here's where my brother and I can go and find the same *National Geographics* from 1910 right there on the same shelf where they've been since before we were born. Here's the venerable rug, the creaky dark wooden stairs with depressions worn in them from Alexis's shoes, the luminous portrait of Katrina at the foot, portraits of my mother and of Violet from when they were rival beauties a half century ago. There's the gas stove in the kitchen that you light with a flint. Here's the long table, polished to a sheen by decades of elbows. Alexis's paintings: Christ's agony on the cross, voluptuous nude women. The furniture, dust molecules intact. The piano, untuned now for close to fifty years, still sinking into the floor. The aroma, even more distinctive than the aroma of my mother's house. It's . . . reassuring.

Tommy and Paulie and Bobby are working on the rest of the house while I concentrate on Mom's study. This will take many days. Before I'm finished, I will handle every book and every piece of paper in this room. I'm glad that this rarefied and labor-intensive archaeological job will be my exclusive province while the men are hauling freezers and mattresses and old tires. But that doesn't mean it's easy. This is a little like Outward Bound, that program where they take problem kids, or kids who wouldn't know a tent-peg from a tire-iron or whose fathers think they're sissies, and send them off into the wilderness with a penknife, a compass and a toothpick. Only this is Inward Bound, boot camp for sentimental cripples. I'm the biggest sissy of them all, and I've been airlifted and dropped directly into a swamp of snares, a morass of sorrows, armed only with whiskey and a trash bag.

Danger lurks everywhere, springs out at me from books, envelopes, boxes, drawers. I'm assaulted by the contents of an innocent-looking file folder, one of the first encounters: Inside it are my mother and Mike's love letters from the early days. I read a few. Their voices are clear, lucid, vibrant. Two songbirds in perfect pitch: Mike is courtly, attentive. My mother basks in his focused love. She's witty, erudite. Their letters are full of newsy tidbits, sharp observations and humor, writers writing to each other. The closing lines are poetic, composed, ardent.

Nope, I think. I'm not going to keep these or even read any more. Out they go. I think maybe I'll survive: caught my first rabbit with my bare hands. If I can toss out their love letters, I can toss out anything.

And I do. I fill trash bag after trash bag. I throw out a huge box of notes, drafts and manuscript material from the Audubon book. I throw out old computer disks and slides. I cull while I'm doing it, setting choice stuff aside, but I'm very, very strict with myself. There's one major exception: books. I don't throw away a single book. That would be a desecration and a sacrilege. I keep a few, pack all the rest into boxes for Bobby: Antique encyclopedias, dictionaries, zoological and botanical compendiums, concordances, pharmacopoeia, biographies, history, old medical texts. God, the range and depth . . . :

Here's her bulletin board, things she's pinned there because they amused or intrigued her: a picture of herself in *Murder in the Cathedral*, a photo of Baryshnikov in flight, clipped from a magazine; a cartoon from a long-ago *New Yorker* showing the Grim Reaper standing at a woman's door, saying, Relax, I've come for your toaster; a quote from Mark Twain, in her own handwriting, about how the fleets of the world could float in spacious comfort on the innocent blood shed in the name of religion, and one of my all-time favorites, an utterance by Genghis Khan in 1226, neatly typed out by mother: *The greatest happiness is to scatter your enemy and drive him before you, to see his cities reduced to ashes, to see those who love him shrouded in tears, and to gather to your bosom their wives and daughters.* This bit of paper has been there so long it's brittle. I pull out the pins with care and tuck it into an envelope in the "save" box. I want it for *my* bulletin board.

Oh, God. What's this? A box of journals. The spines say: "Vinalhaven, 1972, 1973, 1974," and so on. It's years and years of a log they kept of visits to Mike's family's rustic little summer place on an island in Maine. I pull one out. Mom's handwriting alternating with Mike's. Mike inventories repairs, unreliable plumbers, stolen firewood. My mother writes about what flowers are in bloom when they arrive, what some salty Yankee said on the boat on the way over, the local gossip. They write about sharing a cocktail, what the sunset was like, what they cooked for dinner. Their distant voices, long-ago summers and happy times, rise up from the pages. I slam it shut. Nope. I could wander forever here, like Dr. Livingstone. Out they go. Well, not quite. I grab a random handful, two or three. The rest go.

Here's something hilarious. I'll definitely keep this. It's a piece written by a woman who rented my mother's house for a year or so when
Mike and my mother were still editors at *American Heritage*. The woman
was developing a theme, probably as an article for a women's magazine,
on beauty tips. And not just any old beauty tips. She was talking about
looking beautiful for the Lord. Hair, makeup, nails, skin moisturizers,
perfumed bubble baths, all for the Lord. And she was serious. She was
also an atrocious writer. The woman had left it behind when she vacat-
ed. Big mistake. My mother fell on it with glee, made copies and put
withering comments in the margins. Like: *No mention anywhere of looking beautiful for her husband* . . .

Uh-oh. Danger! Grizzly bear! Here's the box of hundreds and hundreds of letters written to my mother by friends after Mike's death.
Tearing of hair, gnashing of teeth. I happen to know my mother
answered every single one. Out, out, out.

Here's a letter my mother wrote to someone, talking about a mutual friend who was, in her words: *". . . gone into Alzheimer's."* A letter from
my mother's sister, complaining about a family house my mother had
sold over fifty years before and how my aunt had wanted to keep that
house. Out.

All the while, I'm looking, looking, with fading hope, for that photograph. The room is actually beginning to empty. Soon I will have run
out of places to look. Bobby and Paulie, grunting and heaving, haul
away the heavy boxes of books, the wooden tables and shelves Mike
built for my mother, Mike's computer, the bags and bags of stuff I'm
throwing out. Down the stairs and gone. Tommy labors in the basement,
a worse job than the Augean stables Hercules had to clean. I look out
the window every once in a while and see him come up the basement
stairs to the lawn, filthy and sweaty, a bandanna covering his nose, carrying some nightmarish load.

Everywhere in my mother's study, thousands of notes, typed or
scribbled—research, ideas, references, inspirations, ideas, ideas, ideas. This
is how it is. Ideas fly by; you try to net as many as you can. Out of the
ones you manage to net and pin, only a handful will ever get your attention. And out of the ones that get your attention, a fraction will make it

all the way through the process of creation and see the light of day. Unfinished work, unstarted work, every idea a magic door, a possible reality, so many that you would have to live for a thousand years to even get started on them. And now, out of these countless scraps of my mother's that have survived thus far, a random few will escape the trash bag. It's the best I can do. It's all I can do. I set aside a big bound journal, dense with her handwriting and covering years, and a little dimestore spiral notebook with Edmund Wilson-like observations of what she saw on the streets and subways of New York.

Then, pay dirt! In an envelope tucked in a book, I find a photo with a caption, clipped from a newspaper: *A kiss for the bride from United States film director John Huston after yesterday's 'hunting wedding' in County Kildare.* The newsprint is as flimsy as old Kleenex, and the picture is slightly grainy, the way newspaper pictures are, but it's fine. Just fine. There's Durant, grinning directly into the camera, a hint of mockery around his eyes that only someone who knew him well would be able to see, my mother ecstatic and lovely, Huston kissing her sweetly on her left cheek. There's a lush spring bouquet on her arm—I think I see tulips and lilacs—and she's wearing a pin, a diamond and sapphire horseshoe, which, at the very moment that I'm looking at that picture, is in her wallet in her basket in her room in Vacaville, California. If I don't find the big glossy original, I have this. I handle it as though it were a Dead Sea scroll. It gets its own envelope and goes directly into my suitcase.

And then I fall through an innocent-looking layer of brush and leaves into a pit of sharpened stakes. I find an old FedEx envelope. Papers inside. I dump them out: AUTOPSY REPORT, MICHAEL HARWOOD. Jesus fucking Christ! While my mind shouts *No!* my hands perversely unfold the paper and I look: *Male, Caucasian, age 55 . . . eyes open, fixed and staring . . .* Why the hell do they put in details like that?

I have no idea my mother saved the report, and now it bobs to the surface in all its clinical ghoulishness. I think of Mike's voice in his journal in the months, weeks, days and hours leading up to the surgery. Mike's voice, abruptly silenced. A brief cold interval, then: *Male, Caucasian, age 55 . . .* Mike traveled with my mother to San Diego to keep his appointment with the bone saw and the steel table. *The other side of the line.*

I wad it up. Enough of you.

There are other papers in the old FedEx envelope. Odd, mismatched scraps. I look. Mike's handwriting. Wobbly sometimes, letters repeated here and there. Mike coming out of the anesthesia. Believing he'd made it. Making jokes, asking questions, answering questions. Oh, God. These are the notes he wrote in the I.C.U. when he had the respirator down his throat and couldn't talk. Eleven days' worth. Some to the doctors, some to my mother. Even crueler: The silence came after these.

No. Absolutely not. I take Mike's notes and the autopsy report, go downstairs, put them in the fireplace and light a match. I watch the slim finger of flame rise, the papers catch, curl and blacken, the smoke go up the chimney. Disrespect? Desecration? Not in my book. Fire transforms. Matter combines with oxygen and becomes energy. Pain and sorrow have been trapped as matter in the form of those papers long enough, under the layers in my mother's study, leaking like buried plutonium. No wonder she never got over his death. Now they're set free. Up the chimney, out into the universe. I consult the image of Mike in my head as I do it. Mike, do you approve?

The image says emphatically: *Burn, baby, burn.*

I never find the big glossy photo. It's gone, solid gone, and I empty that room down to the last paperclip. She obviously threw it out, along with the erotic journals. But I do find a rich stash of her lost writings in old-fashioned file boxes—heavy cardboard, green watermarks, metal latches like old suitcases. It's like opening a pirate chest in a hokey movie, beams of light bouncing off gems when the lid is lifted. Inside are folders, neatly marked, everything done in the writerly way of yesteryear—manual typewriter, fine onion paper, carbon copies of her stories: "The Soul of Mrs. Gurney," "The Hunting Knife," chapters from her never-finished third novel, poetry, the "Yours in the Flag" series—and, impossibly, a short story I didn't know about: "The Scouts."

Isn't this the ultimate fulfillment of every collector's fondest hope? To find an actual hitherto-unknown piece of work by a departed artist? A concerto never played, a sketch never seen, a play never staged, a manuscript never published? The artist speaks, comes back from the dead.

This isn't just any artist, either. This is my mother. And if you don't believe that Alzheimer's is the equivalent of death, try living with it for a year and a half. It's worse than death. In the long interval before actual physical death, the afflicted person is insidiously replaced by an imposter. And you yourself, in protracted up-close-and-personal daily contact, also become a grotesque parody of what you once were. And you lose your memory, too. You develop a sort of amnesia of a particularly cruel variety: You can't remember the whole person, the pre-dementia person. Oh, you can *remember,* but the memories are stuck behind heavy soundproof plate glass. You can't get at them. You can't feel them.

I've read and reread her novels. I just about know them by heart. Reading them helps conjure her as the whole person and ferociously good writer that she was, but I've been reading them for years and years, since long before Mike's death, before her slide into despair, before Alzheimer's, before our terrible eighteen months. I need something new to bring her back to life. The other things—her unfinished novel, the two other stories, are almost new because it's been so long since I've seen them. But this? A story, fresh and uncracked?

I put the file box next to the bed. I'll read "The Scouts" tonight.

The house is emptying fast now, the momentum accelerating, the last sand running through the hourglass. Remaining bits of furniture disappear around us and under us, poof, vanishing into history. We are down to two chairs in the dining room. The table is gone. The box spring under the mattress I'm sleeping on is gone; tomorrow morning the mattress and my mother's bedside table and lamp will go. I pack two big boxes with her clothes, which still smell like her and make sorrows and memories bloom in my poor head while I work. The rest we haul to the thrift shop, a melancholy load, things she won't be needing in Vacaville, or ever again—evening dresses, coats, shoes. Boxes and boxes of shoes.

We are just about out of time. The new owners come tomorrow to take possession. There's one big job left: dozens and dozens of framed family photographs. This is a dilemma. What the *hell* do we do with them? Packing them for shipping so glass and frames won't be damaged, some of them fairly fancy, is out of the question, but we're not quite steely enough to just toss them. By now it's triage. I take scissors and screwdriver, start breaking glass and wrenching wood, pop the photos out. Glass and frames discarded, great-uncles, grandfathers, girls in long skirts on porches or on trips to Venice a hundred years ago go into boxes. Now we're really moving. A pile grows by the front door, everything we haven't sold or thrown away, to be sorted, separated, packed, mailed to ourselves, friends, Mike's family. We'll take it all up the hill to André's tomorrow—the last place we can be safe, the last bit of land before flight—and finish there.

That evening, on the mattress on the floor in my mother's room, I read. The story starts on a full moon rural summer night with a woman watching dreamily from an upstairs window while her two young kids run and tumble in the silvery garden and yard below. Her farmer husband captures the kids and puts them to bed.

> . . . *Lillian had soft, fat arms and shoulders and white, heavy legs, and her flesh rolled up from the open neckline of her blouse into the deep, soft creases of her throat. She had set her hair, clamping it flat to her head with criss-crossed bobbypins. The exposed contour of her skull seemed too small for her ponderous body . . . She took a grape soda from the refrigerator, drank down one or two swallows, and spiked the rest with vodka from a bottle in the cupboard under the sink. Then she crossed the kitchen and pressed against the screen door.*
>
> *"Lordy lord. What a pretty night."*

Lillian and her husband are out in the yard enjoying the moonlight when an old Chevy drives up. They have a visitor.

> *Lillian's younger brother came around the corner of the house, tall and bony, walking as he always did with slouched intensity, his arms slightly flexed, like a wrestler coming into the ring. There was a twitch to the articulation of his right hip. It had been smashed when Donnie fell from the back of a moving army truck and was hit by the next truck in the convoy. The corner of his mouth was held down in a wry grin where an indifferent intern had sewn him up after a fight in a roller-*

skating rink. His face and torso were zig-zagged with fine, fil-
igreed scars from the glass of shattered windshields, and on his
upper arm there was a puckered burn where Donnie had
effaced a tattoo with a lit cigarette, on a bet. He had soft,
damp, querulous eyes with long black lashes.

"Hey," he said, grinning at his sister. "Hey, fat girl."

She made a mild pass at his cheek, as if to slap him. "Don't
get fresh. I'll fat-girl you."

Donnie asks Lillian if she wants to take a "run into town." Her tired
husband resignedly lets her go, but says he doesn't want no trouble.
Lillian rushes into the house, pulling out her bobbypins. She fluffs up her
hair and puts on lipstick and she and Donnie roar off into the night . . .

I read the story. Then I read it again. It's late when I finally put it
down. The neatly typed pages of wicked fiction about a quasi-incestuous
brother and sister on a late-night mission almost cover up the pencil
scrawls on the painted surface of the bedside table.

My mother had started writing on walls and furniture during her
last year in the house. Names, dates, appointments, reminders, questions
to herself. Memory was slip-sliding away, and she was desperately trying
to catch it by the coattails, to stay in the land of the living. And what she
wrote tells the whole desperately sad story: *Call Mr. Reed Monday re:*
check and prize. Priority mail! Dr. Karn: What take for stomach settle and cheer-
up?? Tell him stomach NOT state of mind! El-Belle—birthday? When? What
year born?? Before I turn off the light I get up and fetch a sponge and a
can of cleanser and scrub the ghostly writing off the table. I don't want
some auctioneer looking at it, shaking his head and thinking: poor crazy
old woman. And now only the strong, clear voice of the person who
wrote that story will be here in the room with me. My mother's room,
my mother's voice. The crack under my brother's door at the other end
of the hall is dark now.

I lie in bed and listen to the house. Take a virtual tour in time and
memory: Here's the front hall, Mike, so young, extending his hand the
first time I met him. The living room, my mother and Durant scuffling,
her cry: *You don't want me.* The same room where she and Mike eventually got married. The basement, my brother's sick dying puppy con-

fined there before we took it to the vet to be put to sleep. My mother sitting on the stairs to the bottom floor, holding me on her lap, hugging and comforting me while I cry over a cat killed on the road out front. The old kitchen on the bottom floor, my father sitting at the table on a rare visit, in 1960, a cup of tea in front of him, telling my mother and brother and me that Violet was pregnant. The guest room at the end of the hall, hot teenage sex. The stairs, creaking, middle of the night, my brother *carrying* a girlfriend to one of the top floor rooms. Neil having a midday martini with my mother in the room on the bottom floor that would be Mike's study twenty years later. The dining room, my mother's typewriters and papers all over the place when she wrote her first book in 1962, then in 1996 when she wrote her last.

I drowse. To think that this is the last night Tommy or I will spend in this house. Unless something really peculiar happens. Unless . . . unless civil war breaks out. Martial law declared, Connecticut borders closed, only emergency planes and vehicles allowed in or out, we're sorry, state of emergency, there's nothing we can do until the governor lifts the ban. Pending real estate deal cancelled. Brother and sister live on in empty house, hardly any furniture, he takes the bottom floor, she takes the top floor, they run into each other in the kitchen on the middle floor every couple of days or so . . .

. . . *Yep, they were kinda bitter for a while there, then after a few years they pretty much settled in, he got a job selling paint, if I remember right, and she just sort of went way out there, running around town in her mother's old clothes, all dressed up or sometimes going to the store in her nightgown, telling anyone who'd listen she was a writer and such, saying the brother was a writer, too, but he'd just shake his head and go off to work in his old car, the rent-a-car they never gave back, supporting 'em both, driving all over the state. They coulda left finally when things quieted down but it was pretty much too late and they just stayed where they were, besides, he was working steady, the company, Masury I think it was, headquarters over there in Waterbury, gave him a promotion. Then the war broke out in California and they emptied out all the nursing homes, shipped the mother back to live with 'em; the mother's still alive, old, real old, 102 or somethin' like that, and the kids ain't exactly spring chickens neither, both of 'em pushin' late seventies now, they all live there in that old house together, all packed full of junk now so you can't hardly walk in the door, they go for a Sunday drive once in a while over t'New Milford, he don't talk much anymore, but Jesus H.*

*Christ she talks all the goddamned time, you can't shut her up, and the mother,
she just rides in the backseat and don't say nothin' at all 'cept to once in a while
ask for Mike, he was her husband, died about thiry-five years ago. A real nice
fella. A few folks around town still remember him . . . Christ, yeah.*

We're awake early. Our forty-five years will be up in a few hours. The bar-
barian invaders will occupy the house at noon sharp, and the countdown
is on us. The lamp, the table and the mattress I slept on vanish, Bobby and
Paulie hauling away the last load of stuff. Handshakes, farewells. With
Bobby, anyway. We tramp up and down the stairs, up and down, carrying
boxes, piling them by the door, then out to the car, stuffing it, backseat,
trunk completely packed. Old family friend comes, grunts and sweats
alongside us, doing the final cleaning, our voices bouncing and echoing
in the naked house. We mop, sweep, vacuum, scrub. Real estate agent
appears at 11:30, outrider sent ahead by invaders. At noon sharp the new
owners are in the driveway with a van, waiting, we are cramming the last
things in the trunk, backing out the door with the vacuum cleaner, sucking up our dusty footsteps as we retreat. My final view of the inside of the
house is the front hall, handsome black-and-white checkerboard floor, put
there by my mother in 1956. When Mike went to San Diego, I had a
dream—I really did, this is true—and the dream was that I was Mike,
looking at the hall from this exact angle just before I shut the door, and
knowing it would be the last time I ever saw it.

André is planning on living in his house for the rest of his life. I'll burn
it down before I'll ever sell it, he's said. He's not yearning for some other
place. He likes the crows, the churchbells, the gray Novembers. He's
lived in other places, but never very far away or for very long. He's
home, for keeps, dug in for the duration, embraces it. André will be an
old man in that house, and the display of a circa-1890 wooden sled with
rusty iron runners, snow shoes, and a pair of antique leather boots placed
on a shelf over the attic stairs by Alexis in perhaps 1947 will still be
there.

   Alexis was my special pal. He knew me from the moment I was
born. Talking about what it meant to have artistic gifts and the impor-

tance of not wasting them, Alexis once said to me: *One becomes cognizant of an obligation.* When I was in my early twenties, and Alexis was seventy-two, and it was about three years before his death, we stood out in the driveway together on a clear night, looking up at the stars. We talked about space travel. He said he was sure I'd get to go to the moon, that I'd live long enough to do it. I am sure of it, he said in his deep Russian voice. You have *time* in front of you, he said to me, shaking his fist at the night sky. *So much time!*

Tommy and I go to the Chernov house, once our second home, now our only home here, spread out what needs to be sorted, packed, sent. I find a little snapshot of the view from the back deck of my mother's house: the river, the mountain, a layer of mist floating like a long pale chiffon scarf over the valley. I also find an envelope with my name and address on it, in my mother's handwriting, complete with stamps. I put the picture in and mail it to myself.

We finish in the late afternoon. Each of us will carry one item with us onto our respective flights—artwork, by Alexis, from my mother's house. One is a superb fantasy dreamscape in watercolor, the other is a pencil sketch of my mother, very young, in profile, emphasizing her elegant nose, probably done during her fling with Alexis ages ago. I'll take the dreamscape, Tommy will take the portrait. We agree that sometime later maybe we'll trade. Tommy meets with the real estate agent: The check is put in his hand. We all go out for a farewell dinner, with André, his wife, a few other good old friends. Jolly, noisy, drinks, a huge, impossible job behind us. We will leave tonight. We will drive to Hartford, spend the night in a motel near the airport, and take to the sky at dawn.

We go back to André's house after dinner. Our bags are in the trunk of the big Chrysler rental car. We get in. The doors shut with a muffled ultra-modern *thoomp,* so different from the heavy clank of car doors in the old days. My brother turns the key. The dashboard comes alive with beautiful amber, green and red lights and LED readouts, the big engine purrs. The electronic windows roll down, smooth as the portals on the Starship *Enterprise.* Good-byes all around, friends standing in the darkness outside the car, in the sweet Connecticut May-night air. Somebody says: *Good-bye, Cooneys.*

The windows glide up. It's an airtight, soundproof seal. Climate-control air blows gently, the big tires roll down the long potholed dirt driveway, the Chrysler's luxury suspension smoothing it to the asphalt of a runway. One hundred feet, a right turn, another hundred feet. The powerful beams of the halogen headlights pick out shapes ahead: tomb-stones. Instead of turning left, we glide straight forward on the road that wends its way through the cemetery, around and out the other end. There's the big tree where Tommy and André carved their names. We can't quite make out the letters, but we see the darkish place on the trunk where we know they are.

I know where Miss Wood's stone is: a right on the road, then about twenty paces west. Way to the south of Miss Wood is Miss Janie, and far-ther south, closer to the church and the really old stones from the 1700s, the grave she made the little children stand over when it was a black hole on a long-ago spring day. Way at the north corner, the far end, a boy my brother knew, his age, dead of measles in 1951; a few steps away, a boy we both knew, older than us, a handsome smart teenager, killed in a car crash in 1959. Tommy and I saw the aftermath of the wreck, cops and ambu-lance, whirling lights, a crowd, dark snowy night, Dad driving us home. We begged to stop and look; he said absolutely not. And there, Yulya, a glamorous buxom singer, Hungarian, wife of a friend, pulled a bright red lipstick out of her purse once at a party at my mother's house when I was about ten, gave it to me, cancer, 1960. Over there, Gretchen Osborne, teenager, car crash. And there, Roddy Gregor, twenties, car crash. And there, Katrina Chernov: old age. The Chrysler accelerates down the smooth black strip of paved road that intersects the tombstones.

The console lights glow bright with a surge of power. The wheels retract, tucking themselves in so that the outer skin of the craft is smooth, frictionless. The craft hovers for a moment, then it rises, humming, slowly at first, above the rows of stones and crosses, above the big trees, the gray church, the black road. Another surge, a slight moment of turbulence, the lights of the console glowing brighter again with the extra power needed to break free of the heavy gravitational field. The stones and trees are lost in the dark distance below. Then the hills of west-ern Connecticut recede. The craft rises free and fast. The vast horizon of the earth begins to curve, and the stars, unobscured by atmosphere, grow huge and shine like diamonds. Coordinates are entered, console lights twinkle acknowledgment.

Warp speed. In the amber and green illumination, the tired faces of the brother and sister smooth out, grow younger.

"Music?" says the brother.

"Excellent idea," says the sister.

Sunset, children.

The Hotel California

My mother had a guy for a while. His name was Doug, and he arrived at Sheffield House not long after she did. I spotted him immediately on one of my visits. At first I thought he was another visitor. That's how normal he looked. He was wearing a coat and tie, and had a big photograph album under his arm. He looked cheerful and intelligent and youngish for that place—late sixties, maybe early seventies. And not at all bad-looking. Outside his room was a photo of him with his wife. She's the one who put him away. Putting away a spouse is, I think, about ten times harder than putting away a parent. The guilt and sense of betrayal are much worse. There's that old till-death-do-us-part thing.

But Doug's wife did it. And he immediately became the number one Eligible Bachelor of Kingswood Court. Pretty soon he and my mother were eating together every day. When Mitch and I visit, or when Tommy and I visit, we sometimes stay for dinner, a highly surreal experience. During the Doug era, we sat with him and my mother and their regular tablemate, Ken, the skinny nerdy scholarly-looking guy who didn't even have any gray hair. Ken talked if you talked to him, and was friendly, but painfully diffident, and he never initiated any conversation. Doug was eager to tell stories from his past, and he told them well. He had a repertoire of three or four good tales. When he'd gone through them, he'd tell them again. And again.

He responded really well to conversation with me and Mitch or me and Tommy. He was a good listener and responder. A light of sorts would go on in his eyes, old circuits would be reawakened. He'd crack little jokes, fool around at the table in a fun way, put his napkin on his head, make faces, and my mother would laugh. I watched them play peek-a-boo through a hanging plant once, and on one of my visits she asked me if I'd met "Douglas," using his full name in a fond possessive way. And Doug seemed to remember us—our faces, anyway, if not our names or who we were—from visit to visit.

Gradually, though, jolly cheery gregarious Doug grew sad. I'd look for him, and find him in the TV room, in a reclining chair, staring into the middle distance, face glum, arms crossed. I'd call out his name. Sometimes he'd respond, and wave back. Sometimes he'd just look at me. On the next visit, he might be more like his old self, and then on the next, depressed and remote again. Soon the staff had him eating at a table by himself. I asked why, and they just said it was better for him and everyone else. He'd been, evidently, a bad boy.

Then he was gone. Moved to another facility. He'd "graduated" from Kingswood Court after only a year or so. I asked one of the staff people for details, and she said he was just too big and strong for them to control. I don't like to think of what his life might be like now, of what's being used to "control" him.

This is what happens. They're very, very good at what they do, but as the disease progresses beyond the scope of their ability to care for you and keep you from making life impossible for the other residents, the process fast in some people and slow in others, then you must move on. I'd like to know where he went. I'd like to go and see him, if it's not too far away. Because I'm really, really grateful to Doug. I have no idea of the extent of his and my mother's little flirtation, but on one of my visits, as I came down the hall, I heard something coming from her room that I hadn't heard since Mike was alive: a single explosive two-note ascending laugh of sharp delight, her signature laugh when someone said something really witty. It had been so long since I'd heard it that I'd forgotten it. Doug was standing in the door. I don't know what he said, but it must have been great, because I heard that laugh.

I know she wouldn't remember Doug if I asked her about him. That's merciful, anyway. What's also merciful is that she doesn't mention Mike anymore. Or Connecticut. Terribly sad, but merciful. For her, and for me.

When we first put her in Sheffield House, we held our breath like people driving a truckload of nitroglycerine over railroad tracks. The trouble had started just about on Day One at the Hostel. Why should it be any different at this place?

But it was. The days went by, and then the weeks. Our calls to the staff got us statements like: "Oh, she's doing just great." "She's fine! Stop worrying!" The difference, of course, was that they specialize in dementia, know what they're doing. They know how to divert, occupy, soothe. They apply specific techniques. We found out that on the day we took her there and fled like thieves, they immediately got my mother involved in a balloon-toss game. It sounds ludicrous, but it worked. Diversion, diversion, distraction.

There's a large staff, and it seems as if one of the criteria when they're hiring is that the applicant must be kind and compassionate. Sociologically, Vacaville falls between big city and small town, so there's a large pool of potential staff people but none of that hard, big-city taint. It's a tough job, though, and the pay is not exactly lavish. People do burn out and move on pretty quickly. Residents disappear, and are replaced by new ones, and staff disappear, and are replaced by new ones. But still, it works miraculously well. When I went to Connecticut, my mother had been in Sheffield House for about three weeks. By then it was beginning to look as if it was a go. When one of our calls got us a report about my mother holding hands with Doug at an ice-cream social, I practically fainted.

And I was glad it was as far away as driving a quarter of the distance across Nebraska. That meant it would be just about impossible for my perpetual guilt to make me jump in the car and drive there every five minutes. Anyway, they told us that she'd adjust better if we stayed away for about a month.

Not that it's Elysian Fields, or anything close to it. For what it is, it's extraordinary—but that only means that it is, ultimately, a very civilized loony bin. I don't believe that it's ideal for people with Alzheimer's to live with a lot of other people with Alzheimer's. The ideal would be this: You are very, very rich. You are maintained in a special wing of your own home by a round-the-clock, hand-picked and very well-paid staff of professionals. Your family visits you in your wing of the house, goes out into the garden with you or on little expeditions, maybe eats with you occasionally, perhaps reads to you. You are freshly bathed, groomed, well-fed and in your familiar surroundings. But your family does not clean, cook, feed you, do your laundry, give you baths, babysit you twenty-four hours a day, or change your diapers. That's left to the paid professionals, and so your relations with your family are not contaminated by the cycle of exhaustion, resentment, guilt, misery and hangovers that come with that territory.

If you are not rich, but middle-class with an insurance policy (in the U.S.A., anyway), then it's a place like Sheffield House. There, you'll be clean and well-fed, and of necessity, you'll spend many hours confined with a lot of other people and whatever ghosts are in their heads. I'm amazed that it works at all. Alzheimer's is rarely a happy disease. People tend not to go quietly into that particular night. They moan, cry, complain, squabble. Either that or they get completely quiet, sit with their heads in their hands in attitudes of despair. Cognizance and judgment recede, but certain mental structures remain. In an institutional situation, you have a group of people who probably wouldn't have had anything to do with each other when they were whole now thrown together at random. They're losing social skills and restraints, their minds are fractured, and they're not sure where they are or whether they're awake or dreaming. You might think this is a happy state, a reversion to innocence, but it's not. It's a powerful source of irritation. Losing your mind is highly stressful. Each person is coming from his or her own particular version of this condition, and thus equipped, they must relate to one another somehow.

Comparisons are often made between senile people and children, and it's a useful comparison, but the differences are major. Aside from the most obvious difference—that children are cute and appealing and get smarter every day—there's the most important one: Old people are anything but innocents. They have long lives and thousands of experiences, accomplishments, habits and responsibilities behind them, and they're loath to let go. They've also accumulated a load of frustrations and grievances along the way, and even if they can't remember the specific details, ancient mental patterns have worn deep grooves, and most people are stuck there. One person's ancient frustration butts up against another's and creates fresh frustrations. It happens all day long, every day. It's a wonder they don't kill each other. Sometimes the encounters are darkly comic.

On one of our early visits, there's a new resident. She's a handsome woman with a square, deeply lined face and intense angry eyes. She's dressed immaculately, like a career woman circa 1960: Jacket, pearls, stockings, purse on her arm, hair coiffed. She spots Tommy and me and heads right for us.

"I need a ride to the airport," she says briskly, looking at her watch. "My bags are in my room. Let's go."

We demur. "God damn it," she says. "I'm sick of this crap." She looks around with disgust. "He signed up for another twenty years of duty," she complains.

"Who?" we ask.

"My *son,* for Christ's sake!" she says. We're obviously dolts. "Another goddamned twenty years. I'm sick of this crap. I need a ride to the airport."

Later, we're in my mother's room.

"I'd like to come and try living with you," she says to me. "I'm all alone."

"We're looking for a place," I lie. The door bursts open. The woman with the purse marches in.

"He signed up for another twenty years! I need a ride to the goddamned airport!" She glares at my mother.

"We don't have enough food for dinner," says my mother. "I'm going to have to make a list."

And I think: Where does each woman believe she is? And the thought that inevitably follows: *Where do I think I am?*

I'm well acquainted with my own load of frustrations and grievances. To be spinning my wheels in those particular deep muddy grooves, in the shadow land of senile dementia, would be worse than any hell dreamed up by any religion anywhere.

My father once said that old age is an unnatural condition. When humans were evolving, he said, life was pitilessly short. You reached puberty, bred, and died. If you lived to see thirty you were a phenomenon. You didn't live long enough to have a stroke, a heart attack, lose your teeth, get prostate cancer, go senile. Reproduce and get off the stage—that's all Mother Nature wants you to do. My father said this forty years ago, and recent research suggests he was absolutely right. What they're finding out is that the juices, chemicals and hormones that serve us in youth, that foster rapid growth, strength and reproduction, are often the culprits in the diseases and degenerative conditions of age. Nature's dirty little trick. My father got the full experience: His final years were hard, hard. A stroke left his mind perfectly intact but his body semi-paralyzed, his power of speech deeply impaired, though he could still write and play Scrabble. He lived like that for almost seven years. Violet never put him away. She took care of him to the very end. And that is indeed another story.

I remember a John Updike tale wherein the protagonist, a man in his sixties, thinks that he'd better come up with some new tricks, fast, to keep his Creator entertained. There's a brutal pragmatism to the process of superannuation. When we're no longer a conduit for life, life loses interest in us. It's as simple as that.

I disagree with people who say we in Western culture care little for our elderly. If anything, we err on the side of caring too much. We don't (as a rule, anyway) pack up the camp and leave grandpa behind under a tree. We don't set grandma out on the ice because she can't chew walrus hides anymore. We try. However imperfectly and deficiently, we try. Sheffield House and places like it are evidence of that. A piss-poor (if you'll pardon the expression) solution, ultimately, but an effort in the direction of compassion.

I see a time coming quickly when the requirements of everyday life will push us into incompetence and custodial care sooner. There was a while there when modern inventions were manageable for an older person. Telephones were simple. The TV had an on-off switch. Now you have to program microwave ovens and remote-control devices and cable boxes; instructions are bewildering, electronic menus endless, and the paperwork you must do if you're going to stay in the game burgeons out of control: taxes, balance sheets, jungles of forms and insurance claims. The only possible upside to Alzheimer's that I can think of is that you are finally and forever free from having to do paperwork of any kind ever again.

Some of them start drifting toward the dining room an hour before it's time to eat, going to their accustomed places, sitting, waiting. Others need to be fetched and coaxed to sit. Space is made for us at the table. A room full of children eating is noisy. A room full of senile people eating tends to be very, very quiet. They focus intently on their food. The staff knows each person's little preferences. My mother hates raw tomatoes, likes a glass of milk with her meal. Another won't eat potatoes. The staff, mostly young women, are kind and efficient. "Here's your fruit plate, Edna." "George, do you want pickles today? No? How about some relish?" When they come to us—me, Tommy, Mitch—they say, "Would you like juice? Or maybe some iced tea?" The tone and manner are not much different from what they use with the old folks. It's a little . . . disconcerting.

It's mostly quiet, but there are punctuations. An old man's gruff voice loudly complaining about the food, a group of women at another table murmuring in little birdy voices. A woman who's been there since before my mother, the same woman I've seen a couple of times trying to get out the locked exit door and setting off the alarm, lies down on the floor and cries. There are a few mutterings from the other folks, but mostly they go right on eating, forks clinking.

The young staff women carry trays of medications around to the diners. Little paper cups of pills. Some for physical ailments, some otherwise. At first, my mother wasn't on any medication at all. Then she started slapping people occasionally, like the guy she bipped on the head with the flat of her hand a couple of months ago. She'd been adjusting the curtains in the TV room, he objected. So now she's on a fairly mild twice-daily dose of something to keep her from doing that. I'm sad and sorry about this, but there's no alternative. Not if we want her to stay there.

Deirdre, a staff member who must hold the record for length of employment, passes by me with her tray of pills. I make a joke: "Where are *my* pills?" "None for you today," she says, in exactly the same voice she just used to coax a gent into swallowing water with his medication. Another time, I'd discovered a "volunteer" sunflower growing near the bird feeder we put outside my mother's room. Pleased, I told Deirdre about it, then went to get more bird seed. A couple of hours later, when I was getting ready to go, I told her there was a volunteer sunflower growing outside my mother's room. She smiled and said that was great. Later, I realized what I'd done.

There are two women I'm intensely aware of who are not a hell of a lot older than I am. They're in their fifties, and have early-onset Alzheimer's, which tends to move with the speed of a grass fire in a high wind. One has hardly any gray hair. She's smiling and personable and goofy. Another is a quiet little rotund woman, so young-looking I was sure at first she was somebody's daughter. But she's not.

It's an uneasy feeling. I believe I'm a whole person who can say good-bye and walk out the door and drive away in my car and return to my life, but so does the angry woman with the purse. Tommy and I were heading out once after a visit. My brother started to push open the big glass door. An old lady on a sofa in the lobby called to us: "You have to sign out before you leave!"

So even though I was once grateful that the place is so far away, now I wish it were closer—because the visits have become much, much easier. Things have stabilized for now. She's happy to see us, but she doesn't cling or say heartrending things about Connecticut or wanting to live with me or why did Mike have to die when there are so many bastards in the world who deserve to die. She's forgotten that she smokes, so that's ceased to be a problem. I used to have to go through her basket and pockets to confiscate any matches she might have got hold of, to keep her from lighting up in her room, which she did a couple of times. Sometimes she'll say something about her stomach feeling funny, but the staff tells me it's not much of a problem.

I cannot fathom how it is inside her mind and what it's like for her to be there. She has made some sort of accommodation, but it's terra incognita, and it shifts like a Dalí landscape. On one visit, when we were going back to her room after a walk outside, she looked surprised when I opened the door. "Oh!" she said. "This is just like my room at home!" Another time, indicating the room, she told me that her old friend Phil (who lives in New York) had loaned her this apartment while he was out of town.

The bitterest, bitterest sadness for me is knowing that she believed I betrayed and abandoned her. After she'd been there a few months, I found a photograph of me in her room, ripped in half. In another rare completed letter that I found there, this one to Phil, she wrote:

> . . . I sit now in the sun-struck garden at the motel where I'm presently in residence, some fifteen miles from Ellie's. I learned on my arrival that I was not to live with her—and my time is mostly spent here at my lodging in a local boardinghouse. Today, in fact, she took off for a trip to some place or other in a seaside area. So here I am in my strange new surroundings with no other companions than boarders I've met here. And no extra dollars to live on and pay for food, etc.

How can I live with that? Someone tell me, please. How? I know she wouldn't remember writing that, and she might not be feeling that way anymore, but it's a fact that she did feel it, and that moment exists forever somewhere in the infinitely rippling continuum of the universe. It certainly exists in my head. Mitch remembers a sci-fi book where the protagonist escapes from a space ship that's being drawn into a black hole. There's desperation and confusion. In the melee, the scramble to get into the escape pod and away from the doomed ship, he leaves his lover behind. Too late, he realizes she's not on board. And he knows: She believes he betrayed her. Since she's inside the ship traveling at close to the speed of light, where time slows to a virtual halt, he spends the rest of his days knowing that the terrible moment of betrayal is going on and on and on for her, every minute of his life in "normal" time. For her, it's never over, and he writhes under the burden of that knowledge, and will for the rest of his days. In the case of my mother and me, I'm the one trapped on the ship. The moment's over for her, but for me, it goes on and on.

She started writing fiction again for a while, though she didn't know it was fiction. Her friend Joan sent me a letter my mother had sent to her in Connecticut, thinking I might like to see it. I'm glad she sent it to me, but reading it opened up yet another dimension of sorrow. I knew my mother had finally gone where I couldn't follow:

> I've had four-star new information re: "my lifetime." There will be none of this business of living in or around Hollywood—NO!! Will be living anywhere suitable and comfortable right here on the East Coast. No moving to another part of the world, thank heaven!! The next step is to land a brief part in movie in the making. And from there on, act as I wish in choosing roles—Good! Just as I'd like it. And can go back to Connecticut, or wherever lures me on the East Coast—and still have movie roles from time to time in California. And meantime—a hug from Mary. More anon. Love, love—(I miss you . . .)

All of this in her beloved big loopy handwriting. The sorrow is like nuclear waste. No matter where I store it, or how deep, it's going to eat its way through eventually.

We're entering the twilight, and I wish I could be more present before she slips away completely. She always greets me gladly, but she's a little remote. I don't know how much of what I'm seeing is the disease progressing and how much is the effect of the medication they give her to keep her from walloping people. I wish I were rich and could set her up in her own wing of a house. I wish I could heal all her pain. I wish I had a Star Trek Holodeck and could make a perfect three-dimensional recreation of her house, with Mike in it, alive and whole. If they had the technology, I could do it. I could replicate that house and everything in it and around it, from my memory, down to the smallest detail, down to the soap dish in the bathroom and the ripple in the kitchen window-pane. I do it almost every night in my dreams anyway.

I've done fairly well at compartmentalizing reality so that I can function, but every day, at least once, I feel my stomach drop and the ground roll a little under my feet and I think: *Mom!*

There's a lot of talk of possible new cures. Stem-cell therapy and such. And I ask myself: Shouldn't you go down there, get her out, and try to get her into an experimental program? What if she could be restored? Imagine. Uh—sorry, Mom, we sold your house and everything in it . . .

But she's found a fragile sort of contentment. It would be cruel to rip her out of there. Wouldn't it? And I've ripped her enough, haven't I? And if I failed once, I could fail again. Couldn't I?

I got a letter from a kindly woman who'd read an article I wrote about my mother. The woman had an autistic child, and she'd found a body of research citing amazing parallels between autism and Alzheimer's. The culprit, according to what she found, is environmental toxicity of various kinds, which are treatable with chelation and dietary changes. Her five-year-old son, she said, was recovering rapidly. She urged me to check out the information. This is the kind of thing I'd almost rather not hear about. The what-ifs can drive you nearly insane.

I wrote back to her, thanking her, and said:

> *Alas, I fear it's too late for my mother, unless maybe I get very rich very fast. In many ways she's the ideal candidate for the dietary and nutritional changes you describe; what's unfortunate is that so much psychic damage was done by our horrible experience that I don't know if I have the heart or the guts to try again. I'm just now pulling my life back together. That's the difference between a mother-child and a child-parent situation. The elderly parent's pain and grief is so overwhelmingly powerful it derails everything and just about destroys you.*

I read it and think: Well, that almost convinces me. I hope it convinces her.

And what was *my* contribution to her pain and grief? That's one I'll wrestle with for the rest of my days. It's impossible not to feel that I hastened her decline with my ham-handed attempt to save her. It doesn't matter what people say, how much they try to reassure me. I failed her, and I know it. That's just the way it is.

We drive for hours to see my mother. We stay a shorter time than we spend getting there. Sometimes our presence almost seems irrelevant. She'll lie down for a nap in the middle of a visit. We usually tell her a fib when it's time to go: "We'll be right back, Mom." Then we're on the freeway again. It's the corridor of I-80 between Vallejo and Sacramento. Shopping centers, dry golden-brown hills. A long, long way from Connecticut. The setting sun, red and shrunken, distorted by the particulate matter in the air, looks like an artist's rendering of the dying star five hundred million years from now.

She's okay for the time being. And so are we. But inevitably, we'll get the Phone Call, like the one Doug's wife got. It scares me to think about that. It seems right now as if the worst is over, but what the hell do I know?

What I do know is that I've crossed into new territory from which there's no turning back. My mother was essential to me, in ways I didn't even know about before. My fantastic fortune at having such a mother always conferred a feeling of . . . exemption. I felt anointed, as if nothing really bad could ever touch me. That's gone now. And my lens on the world has darkened a shade or two. A beautiful sunny day and flowers blooming? I look at them and think: So what?

My mother will be on my mind every day for the rest of my life. Sometimes I feel as cynical as Mark Twain on his deathbed when he was bitter and bereft of any faith in life. I understand now why people drink whiskey while they're still in their bathrobes. And I also understand just how flimsy is the infrastructure of cognizance, where our reason, memories and identity lie. It's everything, but it's a delicate and finicky synaptic soufflé. Once it falls, nothing will make it rise again.

I'm also sick of hearing myself whine. I'm aware that I'm singing the white middle-class blues here. I could be in a mass grave in Bosnia. I could be on Death Row in Texas. I'm sure someone living in a tin shack in Haiti would really boo-hoo for me. My share of good luck in this dangerous world is repugnantly disproportionate. I know that for a fact, but I still can't help it—we feel what we feel, and it feels as if my life's been punctured and time is hissing out wildly like escaping air.

Once when I was on a jetliner, experiencing that illusion of motion-lessness that you get even though you know you're going six hundred miles an hour, we passed through some clouds. The clouds were just the right thickness so that I could see them, but they weren't opaque and they were right up close to the plane. For a fraction of a second I was able to perceive the jet's actual awesome speed measured against the clouds. Living with my mother's Alzheimer's, I caught a glimpse of the speed of time going by. Time, which is what our lives are made of.

Yes. My understanding increases daily. Of everything, from Shakespeare to Bo Diddley. I know about weary, stale, flat and unprof-itable now, and for sure, I have a tombstone head and a graveyard mind.

Postscript: The phone rings. Mitch answers it. I'm down the hall, so I can't make out the words. I just hear him talking for a minute or so. He comes to my door, his face as expressionless as a bear's.

"Tricia at Sheffield House would like to talk to you," he says and hands me the phone.

Oh, God. Tricia's the nurse. What is it? Is Mom just running low on underwear, or has she hit somebody in the face? Broken someone's nose? *I'm sorry to have to tell you this . . .*

"Eleanor?" says Tricia. "I'm calling about your mother."

"Lay it on me," I say.

"There's been an incident," Tricia begins carefully. "I'm obligated to tell you about it." *Oh, fuck.* I brace myself. "Um—your mother was discovered this morning asleep in a male resident's bed. She wasn't wearing anything except a shirt . . ." I laugh out loud with relief. Mitch, the sly dog, sand-bagged me completely. He's grinning. Tricia is silent for a moment.

"God!" I say. "That's GREAT!" When Tricia speaks again, I can hear *her* relief.

"She's absolutely fine," she says quickly. "I questioned her carefully, and I looked her over. She says she feels great. There's no sign of any-thing forcible or any trauma."

"Well, hey!" I say. "She was sound asleep in the guy's bed. That doesn't sound like trauma to me!"

"It's our obligation to tell the family when there's an incident like this. Some of the more religious family members get very upset over these things."

"Are you kidding? Upset? I'm about as upset as I'd be if you were Ed McMahon calling from Publisher's Clearing House. And we sure as hell don't have to worry about her getting pregnant," I joke. Tricia is young, married, has a two-year-old. She laughs.

"No, we certainly don't have to worry about that!" she says.

"Listen, Tricia. If she's happy, I'm happy. It's as simple as that. Don't worry about anything. If only you could have known my mother back when she was a red-hot babe having love affairs all over the place. Ha!"

"Yes, well, it happens, and when it's over on the assisted living side, no one thinks anything of it, but when it's here in the Alzheimer's unit sometimes some of the staff worry."

"I know. They tend to see them as children. But they're not."

"No," says Tricia. "They're not. They're adults, and they still have desires."

"Indeed they do," I say.

We chat some more and hang up. I hope I didn't sound a little *too* enthusiastic. But I am my mother's daughter. I'm giddy in the afterglow.

Still have desires.

Well, Mike, I say to the image in my head. What do you think of *that?*

And he smiles.

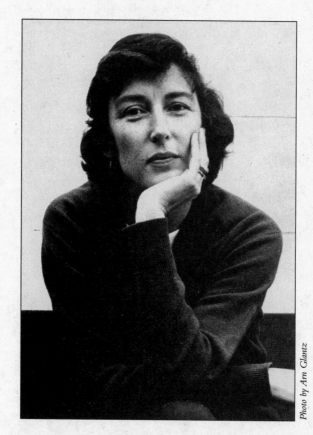

Mary Durant

The Scouts

by Mary Durant

The full moon was so bright, the children ran away at bedtime. They slipped out the kitchen door and across the farmhouse porch and jumped into the silver yard. When Lillian called to them from an upstairs window, the boy, who was seven, and the girl, who was nine, ran among the blue shadows under the trees, darted out the gate to the moonlit precision of the vegetable garden, through the tractor shed and out the far side into the phosphorescent pasture, yipping and tumbling and racing. Lillian leaned on the sill and watched them run.

"You hear your mother?" Harmon hollered from the porch, and the children fell flat in the shining wet grass, pressing their hands over their mouths, panting with fear and pleasure. Their father started after them. When they heard his footsteps crunching through the shed, they broke from cover and ran on across the pasture. Lillian pushed away the curtain that fluttered against her face. "Lordy," she murmured. "Look at that pretty moon."

Harmon strode after the children, seized the tail of the boy's pajama shirt and caught the girl's thin, downy wrist. They dangled and twisted in his grasp, wild with laughter. "That's enough," he said quietly and led them back through the deep moonlight to the house. "Inside. Scoot."

Harmon held the screen door open, and they ran under his big arm into the kitchen. "Lillian, I got the kids. Lilly? You hear me?"

"Ummm . . ." She turned from the upstairs window.

"You hear me?"

"I hear you, Harmon." She moved to the bedroom door as the children scrambled up the stairs. Lillian had soft, fat arms and shoulders and white, heavy legs, and her flesh rolled up from the open neckline of her blouse into the soft, deep creases of her throat. She had set her hair, clamping it flat to her head with criss-crossed bobby pins. The exposed contour of her skull seemed too small for her ponderous body.

In a little while, Lillian came down to the kitchen, stacked the supper dishes on the drainboard and left the pots and pans to soak. She took a grape soda from the refrigerator, drank one or two swallows and spiked the rest with vodka from a bottle in the cupboard under the sink. Then she crossed the kitchen and pressed against the screen door.

"Lordy. Lordy, lord. What a pretty night." Lillian sipped at her drink and squinted toward the far corner of the porch. "Harmon?"

"Yup."

"You there?"

"Yup." He had pulled off his work boots and was sitting on an old army cot set up next to the clapboard siding. One of the dogs started tentatively up the steps, ears down and neck outstretched in supplication. "Git, git!" Harmon snapped his fingers. The dog leaped back and trotted away toward the barns. Harmon lay down, folded the musting pillow and punched it into place under his sun-blackened neck.

"It's a real pretty night," Lillian said.

"Yup."

"You see it?"

"Yup. I see it."

"Wouldn't I just like to run out in that tall grass myself." She pushed open the screen door and stood looking out. "I'd like to go over to Sycamore Park and ride in the speed boat with a whole book of tickets. That's what I'd like."

"Kids in bed?" he said.

"Yup."

"They wash their feet?"

"Yup."

Harmon eased over on the cot and faced the clapboards. His work-day had begun in the cow barn at four-thirty in the morning and would begin again the next day at the same time. Lillian sat down on the steps and looked out across the yard and the still, moon-drenched shapes of the barns and the glistening fields beyond. She hummed to herself, took a few sips of her drink, set down the bottle and re-affixed the bobby pins in a curl over her ear. She patted the other pins appraisingly. In the dis-tance where the highway ran out from town, occasional headlight beams arched across the horizon, and Lillian would stop humming and listen to the rise and fall of sound as the cars passed. One of them slowed down. There was a whine of changing gears on the turning at their cor-ner, and lights bobbled over the pitted dirt road that led to the house. She sat up straight and intent. "Who'd that be?" She listened with her mouth open, eyes fixed on the approaching lights.

"That's a Chevy. Could only be one person."

"Donnie's not the only one drives a Chevy."

"Only one drives a sixty-one Chevy with a broke muffler."

"I can't hear nothing."

"Two bits."

The car stopped by the garage. "Hey! Anybody home?"

"That's him," Harmon muttered. "Mister Shiftless. Mister Bad News himself, in person."

"Hey, Donnie. Hey, yourself!" Lillian called out. "It's Donnie," she told Harmon and pulled herself to her feet, catching her balance against the porch rail. "Here we are! Come 'round back!" she called again.

"God damn." Harmon lay as he was, facing the clapboard wall. "Lilly, I don't want no trouble tonight."

"Mister Worry. Mister Worry."

"Just take it easy. That's all I ask. And I don't want him hanging around late."

Lillian's younger brother came around the corner of the house, tall and bony, walking as he always did with slouched intensity, his arms slightly flexed, like a wrestler coming into the ring. There was a twitch to the articulation of his right hip. It had been smashed when Donnie fell from the back of a moving army truck and was hit by the next truck in the convoy. The corner of his mouth was held down in a wry grin where an indifferent intern had sewn him up after a fight in a roller-skating rink. His face and torso were zig-zagged with fine, filigreed scars from the glass of shattered windshields, and on his upper arm there was a puckered burn where Donnie had effaced a tattoo with a lit cigarette, on a bet. He had soft, damp, querulous eyes with long black lashes.

"Hey," he said, grinning at his sister. "Hey, fat girl."

She made a mild pass at his cheek, as if to slap him. "Don't get fresh. I'll fat-girl you." She grinned back at him. "Where you been keeping yourself, stranger?"

"Harmon around?" He looked toward the porch.

"Where else you 'spect to find me?" Harmon answered.

"Hey there, sport."

"Eh-yup."

"How's it going?"

"High, wide and out of your reach."

Donnie winked at Lillian. "How'd you like a run into town?"

She frowned. "What for?"

"What for?" He shrugged. "A run into town, that's what."

"How come?"

"I'm asking you to take a run into town. That's how come."

"It's not like you take me into town very often."

"Suit yourself." He half turned, as if to leave. "I got the top down."

"Harmon?" Lillian asked.

"Now, wait a minute," Donnie said quickly. "I didn't exactly figure on Harmon wanting to run with me. Looks like he's turned in."

"Right the first time," said Harmon.

"Well . . ." Lillian hesitated. She lifted her face as if she could feel the moonlight against her skin. She stepped to the corner of the house and looked toward the cream-colored Chevy, glinting in the driveway, the roof open to the sky. "Will it be late?"

"Woman, you want a run into town or not?"

"Okay. I'll go. But just for a little while. Okay?"

Lillian hurried back inside, pulling out bobby pins as she went. She combed her hair in front of the mirror over the sink, pushing the curls into place across her forehead and into little puffs on her cheeks. "Ready!" she called, leaning close to the mirror to put lipstick on her tiny bowed mouth. "I'm coming!" She took a deep breath, grimaced, and tugged her skirt down over her hips and stomach. "Harmon, you want the kitchen light on or off?"

"Either way."

She left the light burning and went out on the porch. "Don't you fall asleep out here. You go up and get into bed. I'll be back soon, honey."

"Lilly!"

"What?"

"You take it easy. Hear?"

"Mister Worry. Mister Worry."

Donnie had already gone to the car. Lillian stumbled after him. He stood by the open door to the driver's seat. "Let's go." He dropped behind the wheel, turned the key with one hand while he slammed his door with the other and revved the engine. Lillian lowered herself into the passenger seat. He leaned across her impatiently, yanked her door shut, and the car shot forward, skidding up a wake of dust and pebbles. "Lordy!" she laughed. "Look out, everybody. Clear the track!"

They jounced onto the highway, tires squealing on the turn. Donnie lit a cigarette, inhaling and exhaling meaningfully before he spoke. "Why the hell you have to ask so many questions?"

Lillian bent forward, trying to look at her brother's face, but he held his head to the front and would not look back at her. Then he chuckled and punched at the buttons on the radio.

"Donnie! Now you tell me!" she shouted over the explosion of drums and guitars.

"Wanta dance?" He slurred the car back and forth across the centerline, veering from side to side on the empty road to the beat of the music.

"Donald! You stop that!"

He pulled back into the right hand lane, turned down the radio and smiled as if he were enjoying some sly, secret joke. "How about it, scout? You wanta go scouting?"

"No. No, I don't!"

"Oooo-wheee," he crooned. "I can see him clear and square. Right down the barrel. Right there in that little old sight . . . *tzing.*"

"My God. Who you picking on now?"

"I'm not picking on nobody. He's picking on me. Picking me clean."

"I don't want nothing to do with it."

"Momma, Momma, Donnie won't take me with him. Momma, Momma, make Donnie take me along."

She didn't answer. She sat stolidly, her small lipsticked mouth tight.

"Lilly, Lilly," he chanted, "dressed in yellow, went to the meadow to meet her fellow. Lilly, Lilly, dressed in tan, fell in love with the garbage man . . ."

"You got nothing better to do?"

"Lilly, Lilly, dressed in black, made her drawers from a gunny sack."

She didn't smile. Donnie tilted his head and sucked smoke from the cigarette in the corner of his mouth. "It's that actor over to the play-house that Verna's been going with this summer."

"Verna! You still pestering after Verna?"

"He's leaving at the end of the week. I won't get another night like tonight."

"Christ Almighty. Leave them be. You don't have no claim on Verna. She told me last spring she didn't go with you no more."

"That's mighty interesting," he said dangerously. "So you been talking about me behind my back."

"Once! I saw her once, that's all, downstreet. Hi there, stranger, I said. I don't see you with my brother no more. No, she says, that's done and finished. And that was all. Nobody was talking about you."

"It'll be done and finished," he enunciated, "when *I* say it's done and finished. And it's gonna be finished *my* way."

"You take me home. Right this minute."

Donnie grabbed at her, digging his fingers into the ticklish nerves above her knee. She flailed, slapping at him, shrieking with giggles and pulling at her skirt to cover her legs. "No! I'm going home!"

He pulled his hand away and stepped on the gas. The Chevy bolted forward and streaked between the bright fields and the blue-gray hills. "We're going scouting."

"No, no, no, no!"

He cut the headlights and sped down the moonlit road. Lillian pitched against him. She groped at the dashboard, fumbling across his body for the switch, the wind slashing her hair over her face. He chopped at her wrist and held her away, lazily lifting his shoulder and cocking an elbow into her ribs.

"I promised!" She fought his arm "I promised Harmon."

"I didn't hear you promise Harmon nothing."

"I promised him last time."

Donnie slammed down on the brakes. Lillian collapsed against him, choked with laughter. "You're gonna scare me out of my mind."

"You coming with me?"

She shook her head and giggled wildly.

"Tell me who I am."

Lillian didn't answer. He gunned the engine, gathering speed with jolting, threatening thrusts at the accelerator. He made quick, vicious tickling jabs at her knee, her waist, under her arm.

"DONNIE!" she doubled helplessly.

"Tell me!"

"HAIL, EAGLE FEATHER," she began, through her laughter, thrashing at his marauding fingers.

"Go on," he commanded. "Go on."

"HAIL, EAGLE FEATHER, CHIEF AND SCOUT. KING OF THE INDIANS. BRAVEST OF THE BRAVE. HAIL, EAGLE FEATHER! ALL HAIL!"

He slowed the car to a moderate speed and pulled on the headlights. "That's more like it."

"Christ Almighty . . ." Lillian sat up, raked her hair out of her face and wiped her eyes, catching her breath, breaking again and again into peals of laughter. "Whew!" she cried, wiped her eyes again, pulled at her bunched skirt and twisted blouse and groped for a fallen bra strap.

"We will now," Donnie intoned, "proceed with all fine righteousness on our ordained trail, with a joyful prayer of thanks and goodwill toward everybody. Amen. And of the world to come. Amen and amen." Lillian rocked beside him, her head thrown back, taking deep breaths to stop her laughter. He flicked his cigarette out of the car, and the sparks splashed on the highway behind them.

They came into town on the cemetery road. Gleaming obelisks, polished granite and pearled flights of angels shone through the iron bars of the tall fence. They went on past immaculate rows of quiet houses lit by the amber haze of streetlights, turned right at the parochial school and drove along the green. The stores were closed for the night—the supermarket, the five-and-ten, the drugstore, the Furniture Mart, Cheri's Beauty Salon and Spinelli's Jewelers. At one end of the green, the bronze sorrowing head of Lincoln looked down from its pedestal toward the little wooden bandstand and the memorial Sherman tank at the other end.

Some of the town boys were still cruising in their shiny cars, up one side of the green and down the other. A few had clustered in the empty plaza of the Texaco station, aimless in the summer night, leaning against each other's fenders, smoking, not talking much, watching the street, shifting their loose stance from one leg to another. Donnie blinked his lights.

"Hey, Don!" One of them tooted his horn.

Donnie slowed. "Watch it, you guys. The patrol car's parked in Wheelock's driveway."

The boys howled and cat-called. Somebody barked and ki-yi-ed. "Let's shove off," another one said. Donnie drove on. Lillian turned to look back.

"I didn't see no patrol car at Wheelock's."

"That's right." He glanced in the rear view mirror and chuckled. "Watch 'em scatter."

Lillian looked to the side toward the darkened storefronts. "I don't know who the kids are anymore."

They left town by the river road, passed the deserted ballfield, the gray hulk of the old bleachery and the humming maze of the power station.

"Why're we going out here?" He didn't answer. They turned up a cracked macadam road, Donnie sitting high and tense at the wheel, his eyes dipping from side to side as if scanning the underbrush for danger. The road opened out at the top of the hill into a clearing set with wooden tables and benches. "Hey," she said. "It's the Polish picnic ground."

He maneuvered the car between the weather-warped tables. The headlights picked up a fieldstone barbecue pit, and Donnie swerved to the side. A leafed bough grazed the length of the Chevy. At the top of the clearing, he stopped and turned off the engine. They sat for a moment in the open car, adjusting their senses to the sudden quiet and the moonshadows around them. Lillian looked at him. "You crazy? What d'you want here?"

He got out, went to the rear and opened the trunk, moved a toolbox and the jack, unwrapped the folds of an oil-stained blanket and lifted out a rifle. He raised it and fit it snugly into his shoulder, swinging the barrel across the sky as though sighting a flight of birds. Then he held the rifle loosely against his leg, his shoulders relaxed and rounded.

"Donnie?"

He straightened, stamped his foot and snapped the rifle back to his shoulder. *"Tzing . . . tzing,"* he sang, his mouth pushed askew by the pressure of his cheek against the stock.

"Oh, for Pete's sake!" Lillian said.

"Come on. Let's get going."

"Get going *where?*"

"Hurry up."

"This is the last time. Do you understand what I say?" She slapped the upholstery in rhythm with her words. "The very . . . last . . . time!" She heaved herself out of the car and stood uncertain on the irregular ground. There was a click-clack of the bolt opening and closing, and Lillian knew he had loaded the rifle.

"Come on. You're slowing me up." He went to the edge of the clearing and disappeared into the trees. Lillian labored after him. He had taken a narrow overgrown path where the moonlight hardly penetrated and moved ahead lightly and quickly in the semi-darkness.

"Donnie. Wait up." A sinewy branch snapped back across her shins. She yelped and brought her hands up to protect her face. He waited, catching her arm as she drew close, and dragged her behind him through the interlaced underbrush. They came to an old wall. Donnie sprang nimbly to the other side, set his rifle down and pulled her over the tumbling stones.

"I gotta get my wind." Lillian clutched at him, her feet slipping on slick moss. "Please, Donnie."

"Hush!" He held her around the waist and steadied her. "Shut up that blubbering."

He darted ahead again, leaving her swaying and top-heavy, one hand clutching a frail sapling. Leaves and bark peeled off in her grasp, and she struggled after him, following the moist crackle of his steps. She missed her footing twice and fell sharply on her knees. The tiny thorns of berry vines cut across her ankles, her face, her arms. "Dear Lord," she panted. "Dear Lord."

The trees thinned into scrub and blueberry bushes and sweet fern. She could see better now. Donnie was ahead in the clearing. He'd dropped into a crouch, the rifle close to his chest. He waited until she reached his side. "Keep low," he ordered and hunched forward across an open shelf of rock. At the edge, he lay flat. Lillian hunched after him. "Down!" he told her. She crawled across the rock and lay next to him on her stomach. Stinging lines of sweat ran down her thorn-scratched skin, into her eyes, down her neck and into the bunched roll of her breasts. Around her heart and down one side a creasing cramp swelled and caught when she drew breath. "Lord have mercy!" She rested her wet forehead on her crossed arms.

He prodded her. "See? Now you see where we are?"

Far below the rock ledge was a large, gabled barn, painted red, that had once been a tobacco barn and was now a summer theatre. Donnie clipped a telescopic sight onto the rifle and cradled the barrel in the forked branches of a low scrub oak in front of him. "That's the back exit, from the stage," he said, lining up the rifle with a wide, sliding door. A hooded light over the door shone on a steep flight of wooden steps. At the opposite end of the barn, the wash of the lobby lights fanned out across flowerbeds lining the front walk, over the gravel driveway and up into thickly leafed maple trees. On the far side of a neatly trimmed privet hedge was a parking lot, gleaming with cars.

"See there," Donnie nudged Lillian and pointed down into the dark theatre yard, which lay just out of range of the stage-door light. "See that VW? That beat-up old crate with the ski-rack? You see who's sitting in that little old VW, just waiting to pass it around? You see?"

Lillian's eyes smarted with salt sweat. "I can't see nothing."

"Miss Verna. Sweet Verna."

"I can't see nothing. How do you know?"

"I know, all right. I know."

From inside the barn came the alternate sound of the actors' words and the laughter of the audience. There was a momentary quiet, a final rise and fall of voices, then a rush of applause. The play was over. He turned his attention back to the rifle, steadying it against his cheek, flexing his left hand and soothing it along the cool metal of the barrel. "Any minute. Any minute now."

"What's he look like?" she whispered.

"He puts orange powder on his face and neck and black pencil marks around his eyes."

"No fooling!"

"God's truth."

She wriggled closer to him and slid her arm across his back.

"That's God's truth," he said. "That's what actors do. And this one, fat girl, is a bad actor."

"Yeah?"

"A bad actor . . . get it?"

She giggled. "A bad actor."

"No one'll miss him. One more bad actor."

"One less, you mean."

"That's the ticket."

"One less chicken-dick bad actor," she whispered through her fingers, and they spluttered with laughter. A match flared in the VW with the ski-rack, and a cigarette glowed by the window. "She's smoking," said Lillian.

"If God in his sweet mercy had intended us to smoke, He would have put smokestacks on top of our heads. Amen and Amen."

Lillian shook with stifled giggles and felt his suppressed laughter under her embracing arm and along her side where she pressed up against him. Then he held himself rigid, his muscles tight and primed. The stage door had opened.

"Any minute," he told her. "Any minute. Soon's he gets his pretty face washed." Donnie waited, and she waited with him, pacing her breathing to match his. The cramp in her side rose and fell, and she took shallow breaths to control the little spasms of pain, forcing herself to lie still as she did.

Several people came down the wooden staircase from the stage door and strolled away into the darkness. Car doors opened and closed. A girl in shorts and bare feet came out, sat on the middle step and leaned on her knees. A boy in torn blue jeans joined her for a moment, then wandered off to the front of the building. A woman costumed in an evening dress peered out the door as she stripped long white gloves from her arms. She vanished back into the theatre, and three men appeared under the light.

"That's him. *That's him!*" Donnie hissed. Lillian felt a ripple of anticipation move down his body. She blinked her salty eyes and stared at the stage door.

"The young guy. The one holding the thermos bottle." Donnie ran his tongue over his teeth and released the safety catch on the rifle. "There he is, by God, bigger'n brass. You ready, Lilly? I'm giving him a count of five. Five. Got it? *Five,* and no sooner."

"Five. Yes. Five."

He started counting, slowly and evenly. "One hundred . . . two hundred . . ." Lillian moved even closer against her brother's side, her right arm still clasped across his back, holding him tightly, one heavy leg slung across his. Squirming, she slipped her other hand along his left arm, the arm that held the barrel, until she gripped his wrist. He steadied the sight and continued his measured count. "Three hundred . . . four hundred . . ." At the final count, she counted with him. *"Five hundred!"* Lillian wailed, and heaved up against his left arm, thrusting the barrel skyward just before the rifle cracked deafeningly. The bullet whispered through the tops of the tall trees that surrounded the red barn.

The girl on the steps jumped up and screamed. The men in the doorway ran to her, then they all went down the steps together into the theatre yard and stood close to each other, listening, looking around, speaking briefly and cautiously, their voices lost under the noise of cars leaving the parking lot. In a little while, they separated and moved on.

Donnie rolled onto his back and smiled, the rifle next to him, his eyes black in his moon-blanched face. Lillian, ears ringing, gave a low cry, sighed, put her head down on her arms and fell asleep. When all the cars had driven away and all the lights had gone out at the theatre, he woke her and they started back.